The Role of Medicine

DREAM, MIRAGE
OR NEMESIS?

THE ROLE OF MEDICINE

DREAM, MIRAGE OR NEMESIS?

Thomas McKeown

BASIL BLACKWELL · OXFORD

A shorter version of this book was first published as the 1976 monograph of the Rock Carling Series by the Nuffield Provincial Hospitals Trust.

ISBN 0 631 10701 0

ISBN 0 631 11261 8

Typeset by Cotswold Typesetting Ltd, Gloucester and printed in Great Britain by Billing and Sons Ltd, London, Guildford and Worcester.

CONTENTS

PREFACE TO THE SECOND EDITION

The writer of a controversial paper published in a medical journal soon discovers that those who agree with him write to the author while those who disagree write to the editor. Something of the same kind can be observed in the reception of a controversial book, so that the opposition often appears to be wider and warmer than in fact it is. I do not think I am mistaken in believing that most readers of *The Role of Medicine* were in general agreement with its conclusions, although with so large and complex a theme inevitably there were reservations on certain points, not all of them minor.

However, some people interpreted the book as an attack on clinical medicine, and one or two linked it with Illich's *Medical Nemesis*. A close reading is not required to show that the two books have little in common, except perhaps in the sense that the Bible and the Koran could be said to be identified by the fact that both are concerned with religious matters.

But as 'the more violent the emotions generated by a topic, the harder it is to be rational about it',[1] I should like to remove misunderstandings by clarifying my own viewpoint.

1. I believe that for most diseases, prevention by control of their origins is cheaper, more humane and more effective than intervention by treatment after they occur. As an interpretation of the past this statement is rapidly becoming a platitude; as a prediction for the future I recognize it is still arguable.

2. There are no grounds for criticism of medicine in the fact that medical education, research and practice are based on quite different premises. In their assumptions about the determinants of health, doctors have been under the same misapprehensions as everyone else.

3. The conclusion that medical intervention is often less effective than has been thought in no way diminishes the significance of the clinical function. When people are ill they want all that is possible to be done for them and small benefits are welcome when larger ones are not available. Moreover, inability to control the outcome of disease does not reduce the importance of the pastoral or samaritan role of the doctor. In some ways it increases it.

1. Haldane, J. B. S., *Science and Life* (London: Pemberton, 1968), p. 65.

4. Finally, and on a more personal note, let me add that I do not belong to the small minority of saints, reformed sinners and others for whom physical discomfort is necessary for mental comfort, and if I were ill I should not turn to fringe medicine, acupuncture, transcendental meditation or faith-healing. I should like good medical attention, by which I mean clinical service which combines technical competence with humane care.

Since writing *The Role of Medicine* I have become aware of deficiencies which seemed to justify the preparation of a second edition. Some are related to points raised by reviewers, others to issues which I think I now see more clearly than when I first wrote. The following are among the most important of them.

When assessing the relative importance of different influences on health in the past, I based conclusions on the decline of mortality and made only a brief reference to the treatment of morbidity. This approach was rightly said to underestimate the contribution of clinical intervention, and in a new chapter I have tried to make a more adequate appraisal of medical achievement by considering also postponement of death (from a specific cause) and treatment of non-fatal illnesses.

While most people are agreed about the interpretation of the past,[2] some have questioned my extrapolation to the future: the suggestion that, as in the case of the infections, most non-communicable diseases are more likely to be controlled by removing their causes rather than by intervening in disease mechanisms. I have tried to narrow the area of disagreement by separating diseases into four classes: relatively intractable; preventable, associated with poverty; preventable, associated with affluence; and potentially preventable, not known to be related to poverty or affluence. It is only in the fourth class that there are likely to be considerable differences of opinion about the most effective approach.

I have also considered carefully the suggestion that the conclusion that the main influences on health – nutrition, environment and behaviour – are outside the medical care system has little bearing on the role of medicine.[3] Here I believe it is important to distinguish the role of

2. I share reservations about the reliability of certification of cause of death but they do not affect my main conclusions.

3. 'The major question is to what extent the assessments of *The Role of Medicine* should change the kind of care that the able and conscientious physician gives his patient. Not very much, I think.' Ingelfinger, F. J., *New England Journal of Medicine*, **296** (1977), p. 449.

medicine as an institution from its more limited responsibility for clinical care. I have suggested that in its larger role, medicine should be concerned with all the influences on health, a conclusion that has a considerable bearing on medical education and research as well as on health services. But if medical intervention is often less effective than most people, including most doctors, believe, there is also a need for more critical evaluation of clinical procedures before they are introduced, and for greater emphasis on personal care of the sick (the pastoral role of the doctor). For the large number of patients (among the retarded, the mentally ill and the aged sick) who provide no scope for active measures, the last aim is unlikely to be achieved without a reshaping of health services, particularly hospital services.

I should not like to end this Preface without expressing my indebtedness to my colleague, Professor R. G. Record. We have worked together for thirty-three years, and I have discussed with him nearly every point relating to medical achievement and population growth. If I have been able to avoid serious errors in this wide and treacherous subject, it has been due largely to his sound advice. I am also most grateful to Professor A. G. W. Whitfield who has been kind enough to read carefully the revised edition.

It is a pleasure for me to thank Mrs Eileen Armstrong and my secretary, Mrs Wendy Greenaway, for the care they have taken with the preparation of the typescript.

Peasants and crops, in other words food supplies and the size of the population, these determined the destiny of the age. In both the long and the short term, agricultural life was all-important. Could it support the burden of increasing population and the luxury of an urban civilization so dazzling that it has blinded us to other things? *For each succeeding generation this was the pressing problem of the day. Beside it, the rest seems to dwindle into insignificance.*

—Fernand Braudel, *The Meriterranean and the Mediterranean World in the Age of Philip II*

INTRODUCTION

Speaking of the origin of an idea a historian once remarked: 'It is always earlier than you think'; and certainly it is not possible to name the sceptic who first questioned the effectiveness of medical procedures. But at least from the time of Montaigne, the notion that treatment of disease may be useless, unpleasant, and even dangerous has been expressed frequently and vehemently, particularly in French literature. Molière's *Le Médecin Malgré Lui*, the famous operation in *Madame Bovary* and Proust's account of the psychiatrist's cursory examination of his mortally ill grandmother ('Madame, you will be well on the day when you realize that you are no longer ill. . . . Submit to the honour of being called a neurotic. You belong to that great family . . . to which we are indebted for all the greatest things we know') are examples of the irony and bitterness with which some of the greatest writers have expressed their conclusions about the work of doctors.

Remarkably, considering the eminence of the critics, such views have had little effect on medicine or the public's estimate of it. Perhaps they were not meant to be taken quite seriously; indeed Proust wrote: 'To believe in medicine would be the height of folly, if not to believe in it were not greater folly still, for from this mass of errors there have emerged in the course of time many truths.' Or possibly, being expressed humorously, the criticism incurred the risk of being considered frivolous; it is at least arguable that Shaw's lively Preface to *The Doctor's Dilemma* had less influence than the Webbs' seriously worded essay on a public medical service in *The Report of the Poor Law Commission*. Whatever the explanation, until recently the contribution of medicine to prevention of sickness, disability, and premature death was taken essentially at its own evaluation.

I have no difficulty in dating the origin of my own doubts about the conventional assessment of the work of doctors. They began when I went to a London hospital as a medical student after several years of graduate research in the Departments of Biochemistry at McGill and Human Anatomy at Oxford. There were two things that struck me, almost at once. One was the absence of any real interest among clinical teachers in the origin of disease, apart from its pathological and clinical manifestations; the other was that whether the prescribed treatment was of any value to the patient was often hardly noticed, particularly in internal medicine. (On the latter point, although not the former, the approach in surgery and obstetrics was somewhat different.) I adopted the practice of asking myself at the bedside whether we were making anyone any wiser or any better, and soon came to the conclusion that most of the time we were not. Indeed there seemed to be an inverse relation between the interest of a disease to the doctor and the usefulness of its treatment to the patient. Neurology, for example, was highly regarded and attracted some of the best minds because of the fascination of its diagnostic problems; but for the patient with multiple sclerosis, Parkinson's disease, amyotrophic lateral sclerosis, and most other serious neurological conditions, the precision of the diagnosis which was the focus of medical interest made not the slightest difference to the outcome. If the gifted neurologists had private qualms about the usefulness of their efforts they gave no indication of them, at least in the presence of students. Venereology, in contrast, although it provided the valuable treatment of sylphilis and contributed to prevention of the spread of gonorrhoea, was held in low esteem; so too were some useful surgical procedures including, remarkably, the surgery of accidents, perhaps the most successful of all therapeutic measures. Endocrinology, in which I had been working, was in an intermediate position; through its researches it had reached Burlington House,[1] although its practice was still not far removed from that of the hygienic stores which dispensed rejuvenants on the Charing Cross Road. I concluded that if I were St Peter, admitting to Heaven on the basis of achievement on earth, I would accept on proof of identity the accident surgeons, the dentists and, with a few doubts, the obstetricians; all, it should be noted in passing, dealing mainly with healthy people. The rest I would refer to some celestial equivalent of Ellis Island, for close and prolonged inspection of their credentials.

The opportunity and incentive to consider more deeply what was initially little more than an undocumented impression, came through my appointment to the Chair of Social Medicine at Birmingham. In the early 1940s some senior teachers had come to the conclusion that a medical school located in the industrial Midlands should have a department of occupational health, and an application was made to the Nuffield Provincial Hospitals Trust which was known to be interested in the subject and had made a grant for the same purpose to Manchester.

---

1. At that time the home of the Royal Society.

The Trust offered to finance a chair of social medicine but not of occupational health; so on the sound principle of not looking a gift horse in the mouth the University accepted the grant and changed its intentions. However, one of the attractions of the term social medicine at that time was that each could interpret it in his own way, and I doubt whether the change of title was considered important.

My own association with the new department was fortuitous, to say the least. I had been interested in another post (in the Department of Medicine), when the University, having advertised the Chair twice with disappointing results and presumably at a loss about what to do next, invited me to submit an application. The only requirement, apparently, was that I should be seen and not objected to by Sir Farquhar Buzzard, then Regius Professor of Medicine at Oxford and adviser to the Nuffield interest. I met Sir Farquhar in his rooms at Christ Church at lunchtime; but not for lunch, as I could not fail to perceive from the fact that the College servant was preparing the table for one. For a moment I thought I might find myself in the position of the courtiers of Louis XIV, who attended patiently while their monarch supped singly and in silence. However, the interview was short and scarcely delayed his meal, to which no doubt I largely owe the fact that he evidently raised no objection to my appointment. The background was illuminated further when I eventually took possession of a room in the Medical School, shared previously by the part-time teacher of public health (Dr G. A. Auden, father of the poet) and the lecturer in forensic medicine, and filled with drains, waterpipes, contraceptives, and numerous other objects of forensic and nineteenth-century public health interest. The room also contained the applications for the post to which I had just been appointed. After perusing them I could see the University's difficulty. One candidate included among his credentials that having committed himself to no line of activity he was free to proceed in any; another stated that he had been advised by his doctor to seek lighter work; a third had the misfortune to name a referee who wrote that the applicant did not suffer fools gladly, always an unwise thing to say to a selection committee, since it makes them uncomfortable.

In the Department of Social Medicine the contribution of medicine to improvement in health was a subject of intermittent interest but no detailed research until 1953 when H. J. Habakkuk published an article on the growth of population in England during the eighteenth century. In it he questioned the traditional interpretation, proposed by Talbot

Griffith in 1926 and accepted by most social historians, that the increase was due to a decline of the death-rate brought about by advances in medicine. Habakkuk considered that the medical measures of that period looked insufficient to account for the rise of population and turned to the possibility, attractive to some historians, that it resulted from an increase of the birth-rate which was secondary to economic and industrial developments. Our own view (I speak here also for my colleagues subsequently associated with this work) was that Habakkuk's estimate of medical measures was correct, but that nevertheless a fall of mortality was a more plausible explanation for the growth of population than a rise of fertility. A first paper on this subject (in 1955) was followed by others concerned with population growth in the nineteenth and twentieth centuries, and in a recent book (*The Modern Rise of Population*[2]) I have attempted a comprehensive interpretation of the increase of population from the eighteenth century to the present day. This book was first suggested to me by an Oxford historian, John Cooper, but I did not think seriously of tackling it until 1973, when at a meeting in Pavia I discovered that there was a considerable industry among French and Italian historians working on such unrewarding topics as the decline of plague and inoculation against smallpox in the eighteenth century.

In the meantime I had come to see that recognition of the limited impact of medical procedures was a key which would unlock many doors. My own interest in it was initially, and is still primarily, in its significance to medicine and health services, and this is the theme of the present monograph. To state it simply: misinterpretation of the major influences, particularly personal medical care, on past and future improvements in health has led to misuse of resources and distortion of the role of medicine.

Since this statement may appear to have an affinity with the conclusions reached by Professor Cochrane in his notable Rock Carling Lecture on *Effectiveness and Efficiency*, I must try to distinguish between our approaches. I think of him as an itinerant preacher who emerges at intervals from his Welsh retreat to admonish the faithful for their failure to submit all aspects of their lives and works to scientific appraisal by randomized controlled trials; myself I see as an academic Billy Graham who bears the glad tidings of health for the taking to a grateful people. The distinction will be worth a closer examination.

2. Edward Arnold, London, 1976.

Introduction

In *Effectiveness and Efficiency* Cochrane criticized the organization of medical services and to a lesser extent, or at least more briefly, the direction of medical research. The grounds for his criticism of services were two-fold: many medical procedures and services have not been tested for their effectiveness and a considerable number of those which have been assessed were found to be unsatisfactory; and there are gross inequalities in standards of services, particularly between the 'care' and 'cure' sectors. Although few people are likely to question the last assertion, it should be noted that it was not based on, and probably does not permit or require, the same kind of validation as a clinical procedure. Finally, although the monograph refers briefly to environmental and behavioural influences (the importance of population policy was emphasized in the Conclusions), it was concerned mainly with clinical procedures and services.

What should be observed about this approach is that it does not suggest that there is anything seriously wrong with the traditional lines of health services and medical research, apart from the imbalance in investment between care and cure. Moreover the last is a pragmatic rather than a conceptual criticism. What is said to be lacking is scientific evaluation of measures before they are introduced, and it is implied that if everything were submitted to randomized controlled trials, effective clinical procedures and services would in time appear (an endorsement of Proust's view that from the mass of errors there would emerge many truths).

It need hardly be said that Cochrane's emphasis on the need for critical appraisal of medical measures was entirely justified, and being based largely on his own extensive experience had an impact which no other approach could have matched. Indeed, as noted on the first page of this Preface, our health traditions have had no difficulty in living with criticism from outside; but they are more vulnerable to attack from within, to the suggestion, not that medical activities are misdirected (an unlikely conclusion from a son of University College Hospital who has laboured in the vineyards of the MRC), but that they are not sufficiently scientific. However, I see the exchange as an opening round in a long engagement, in which the premises on which health, and particularly medical activities are based, require to be explored. My own position, in distinction from that of Professor Cochrane, is, briefly, as follows.

Medical science and services are misdirected, and society's investment in health is not well used, because they rest on an erroneous assumption about the basis of human health. It is assumed that the body can be regarded as a machine whose protection from disease and its effects depends primarily on internal intervention. The approach has led to indifference to the external influences and personal behaviour which are the predominant determinants of health. It has also resulted in the relative neglect of the majority of sick people who provide no scope for the internal measures which are at the centre of medical interest.

This book presents the grounds for these assertions, and examines their significance to health services and to medical education and research.

Part One

Concepts of Health and Disease

I

Evolution of Health Concepts

The aims of this book are: (a) to examine the validity of a concept which is rarely stated explicitly but on which medical activities largely rest, namely that human health depends essentially on a mechanistic approach based on understanding of the structure and function of the body and of the disease processes that affect it; and (b) to consider the significance of the conclusions for medicine, particularly in relation to health services, medical education, and medical research. These themes are discussed in the three sections into which the book is divided, the first two concerned with concepts and determinants of health and the third with the role of medicine.

Although the mechanistic approach is predominant it is not the only one which has been taken to improve man's health. In his splendid account of the evolution of health concepts Dubos referred to the dual nature of medicine which resulted from ideas which have been promoted with varying emphasis in all periods down to the present day: health preserved by way of life and health restored by treatment of disease. Both are to be found in the classical tradition:

The myths of Hygieia and Asclepius symbolise the never-ending oscillation between two different points of view in medicine. For the worshippers of Hygieia, health is the natural order of things, a positive attribute to which men are entitled if they govern their lives wisely. According to them, the most important function of medicine is to discover and teach the natural laws which will ensure a man a healthy mind in a healthy body. More sceptical, or wiser in the ways of the world, the followers of Asclepius believe that the chief role of the physician is to treat disease, to restore health by correcting any imperfections caused by the accidents of birth or life.[1]

The preservative approach was certainly in the minds of the social and

---

1. Dubos, R., *Mirage of Health* (London: George Allen and Unwin Ltd, 1960), p. 109.

medical reformers of the eighteenth and nineteenth centuries, and it is to be found in the public health activities which resulted from their efforts and have continued and developed to the present day.

Philosophically the seventeenth century was a turning point in the balance between the two concepts. Galileo had shown that scientific methods were capable of providing a mechanical interpretation of the physical world, and Descartes saw no reason why the same principles should not be extended to living things. He conceived of the body as a machine, governed entirely by the laws of physics, which might be taken apart and reassembled if its structure and function were fully understood. His theories seemed to find confirmation in the first major development in modern physiology, Kepler's description of the dioptric mechanism by which the eye produces the retinal image. This advance resulted from the application of technical knowledge available in second-century Alexandria, but which no Greek would have thought of bringing to the study of the living body. A little later there was an even more dramatic demonstration of the validity of the mechanistic approach in Harvey's discovery of the circulation of the blood, which Descartes, needless to say, warmly welcomed.

In the present context there are three aspects of the hypothesis to be considered: the relation between mind and body; the body interpreted as a machine; and the body controlled as a machine.

The first subject need not detain us, although it has been the focus of endless controversy at the interface between science and theology. Briefly, while Descartes as a scientist could accept a physical explanation for the body, as a religious man he was unable to accept it for the mind; so he found it necessary to distinguish between mind and body, and he introduced what Ryle described as the Category-mistake, the notion of the mind as a ghost in the body as a machine.[2] Temporarily at least, this explanation furnished a reconciliation of sorts between the results of the new science and the traditional doctrines of the soul. However, although this problem has engaged the attention of philosophers and theologians for centuries, for many scientists educated since the First World War I suspect it has scarcely existed. Unencumbered by preconceptions derived from religion or scholastic philosophy, they have never thought of the mind as something which exists apart from the physical structure of the body. Their problems arise mainly from

2. Ryle, G., *The Concept of Mind* (London: Hutchinson's University Library, 1950).

the other implications of the Cartesian hypothesis: the body conceived as a machine and the body controlled as a machine.

There is no difficulty today in accepting that the body can be understood as a machine, of which knowledge has advanced continuously from the seventeenth century; slowly at first, but very rapidly at the cellular level since the nineteenth century and at the molecular level in the twentieth. In parallel with the understanding of structure and function there was an increase in knowledge of disease processes, including, in the case of infectious diseases, recognition of disease agents. It is hardly surprising that the transformation of human health which occurred in the same period was attributed to the new knowledge, and that the improvement in the performance of the body as a machine was assumed to be due to its control as a machine.

However, this is an assumption which must be examined carefully. In the first place it should be noted that in the past three centuries conditions of life have improved more than in any previous period in man's history. For large populations the chronic problem of malnutrition has been solved; some of the most serious threats, particularly those associated with water and food, have been removed from the environment; and for the first time on an extensive scale human populations have limited their reproduction to a level consistent with basic resources. In assessing the contribution of medical measures based on understanding of the structure and function of the body, it is clearly essential to consider the extent to which the advance in health was due, not to intervention in the working of the machine, but to improvement in the conditions under which it operates.

There is another reason for caution before endorsing the conventional explanation for the advance in man's health: the fact that quite a different interpretation must be accepted for the improvement in health of other living things. The brief discussion which follows will be concerned with animals, although many of the conclusions would be equally true for plants.

The key to the riddle presented by the health of living things is the relation of fertility to mortality. Both have evolved through natural selection; but they have not evolved in balance, in the sense that numbers born are restricted with regard for the resources of the environment and the numbers that can survive. A contrary view, that animals limit their reproduction by social and biological restraints[3] was strongly

3. Wynne-Edwards, V. C., *Animal Dispersion in Relation to Social Behaviour* (Edinburgh: Oliver and Boyd, 1972).

challenged,[4] and since it has no relevance to human experience in the past few centuries it will not be considered here.

The alternative, and I believe the more convincing interpretation, suggests that the size of natural populations is controlled by density-dependent mortality. In wild birds and some other animals (Lack mentioned carnivorous mammals, certain rodents, large fish where not fished, and a few insects) the level of mortality is determined mainly by the availability of food. However, there are other animals, possibly many more, in which, although numbers are limited ultimately by food supplies, these limits are not usually reached because population size is restricted by predators, including insect parasites, and disease.[5]

On this interpretation the essential requirements for reduction of mortality and improvement in health of animal populations are (*a*) equating of food supplies and population size, by increasing the amount of food and limiting numbers, and (*b*) removal of other causes of mortality, particularly predators, including in some cases human predators, and parasites.

This theoretically derived programme is in accord with what has actually happened in domestication of plants and animals. Their numbers and distribution are controlled; more and better food is provided: manure and fertilizers for plants, foodstuffs in a variety of forms for animals; and domesticated plants and animals are protected so far as possible from environmental hazards.

Another method of outstanding importance is selective breeding, which has been used with all domesticated animals except the elephant. (Elephants rarely breed in captivity.) This approach has been employed to accentuate characters desired by man, sometimes with side-effects on health from production of pure strains which are less resistant to microorganisms. But cross-breeding has been used to produce hardier stocks by heterosis.

The methods which have been exploited in plant and animal husbandry are essentially population methods which owe little to understanding of structure and function. It is fairly obvious why this approach has been preferred to physical or chemical manipulation of individual plants or animals. In the first place, except in the case of pets and unique specimens such as racehorses and prize animals, man has little interest in individual examples of species other than his own. Secondly, it is

4. Lack, D., *Population Studies of Birds* (Oxford: Clarendon Press, 1966), p. 299–312.

5. Lack, D., op. cit., p. 287.

more economical to deal with large numbers in preference to identifying and controlling single specimens. And finally, a conclusion which is particularly important for human health, population methods are far more effective than individual methods. Indeed, when they are fully applied there is little need for direct intervention, for under favourable conditions the large majority of those born alive remain healthy.

To what extent is it possible to extrapolate from other animals to man? Until the eighteenth century the human situation was analogous to that of animals in their natural habitats; numbers born were greatly in excess of numbers that could survive, and population size was limited by density-dependent mortality. There is no evidence of effective restriction of population growth, either by deliberate control of reproduction or by instinctive restraints of the kind suggested by Wynne-Edwards in other animals.[6] The high level of mortality was due to starvation, disease, and homicide in its multiple forms.

In these circumstances human health provided scope for the methods which led to improvement in the health of domesticated animals. Like other living things, man has been exposed to rigorous natural selection, and the large majority of those born alive are healthy in the sense that they are adapted to the environment in which they live. The primary need is for sufficient food, which requires both an increase in food supplies and limitation of numbers. Man also needs protection from certain hazards in the physical environment, particularly those which lead to exposure to infective organisms. The notable difference between human and other animal experience in relation to health results from ethical restraints which prohibit public control of reproduction. But man is uniquely educable, and can learn voluntarily to limit family size. In this way a self-imposed behavioural change may achieve the same result as the restrictions applied to other animals.

However, the approach to biology and medicine established in the seventeenth century was an engineering one based on a physical model; its consequences are even more conspicuous today, largely because the resources of the physical and chemical sciences are so much greater. Physics, chemistry, and biology are considered to be sciences basic to medicine; medical education begins with study of the structure and function of the body, continues with examination of disease processes and ends with clinical instruction on selected sick people. Medical service is dominated by the image of the acute hospital where the technological resources are concentrated, and much less attention is

6. Wynne-Edwards, V. C., op. cit.

given to environmental and behavioural determinants of disease, or to the needs of sick people who are not thought to provide scope for investigation or treatment. Medical science also reflects the mechanistic concept, for example in the attention given to the chemical basis of inheritance and the immunological response to transplanted organs. These researches are strictly in accord with the physical model, the first being thought to lead to control of gene structure and the second to replacement of diseased organs by normal ones. The question therefore, is not whether the engineering approach is predominant in medicine, which would hardly be disputed, but whether it is seriously deficient as a conceptualization of the problems of human health.

The first two parts of this book are concerned with an examination of this issue. There are at least three approaches which might be taken to assessment of the determinants of human health. One possibility would be to examine, where possible by controlled trials, the effectiveness and efficiency of medical procedures and services, as well as other influences, such as food and hygiene, which contribute powerfully to health. This approach has been employed with great advantage in a limited number of cases; but it presents formidable technical, ethical and administrative difficulties and it is hardly conceivable that within the foreseeable future it could provide a comprehensive appraisal of all the major determinants of health. I have therefore restricted attention to the other possibilities.

Chapter 2 outlines a conceptual approach. It suggests that if we are thinking of disease origins rather than disease mechanisms, the most fundamental division is between abnormalities determined irreversibly at fertilization and those which are manifested only in an appropriate environment. Among the latter there is an important practical distinction between congenital conditions in which the environmental influences are pre-natal and those, including most common diseases in which they are probably post-natal. Although post-natal influences vary greatly in type, it is suggested that it is on their identification and control that hopes for the solution of the problems of the common diseases largely rest. This approach can often succeed in spite of deficient knowledge of disease mechanisms.

The next three chapters present the third approach, an examination of historical evidence; they are based on data for England and Wales which are perhaps the most satisfactory for this purpose. It is shown that the decline of mortality, the main evidence of improvement in health, was due essentially to a reduction of deaths from infectious diseases. (The only non-infective causes which appear to have decreased substantially before the twentieth century were infanticide and starvation.) Chapter 4 investigates the reasons for the decline of the infections, and Chapter 5 considers non-infective conditions which were associated with about a quarter of the reduction of mortality since 1900.

The conclusions concerning the determinants of man's health are brought together in Chapters 6 and 7, which examine man's health experience in four periods: nomadic, agricultural, transitional and industrial. The predominant influences which led to the improvement in health in the past three centuries were nutritional, environmental (particularly control of water and food), and behavioural; the last through the change in reproductive practices which limited population growth. The major influences are reconsidered in the light of the change in health problems which followed the decline of the infections, and it is concluded that in advanced countries health is still determined mainly by personal behaviour and the environment. However, there is this difference, that the influences which result from the individual's behaviour (smoking, diet, exercise, etc.) are now relatively more important than those which depend on action by society. The contribution of personal medical measures remains tertiary in relation to the predominant behavioural and environmental influences.

Chapter 8 assesses medical achievement in relation to prevention of death, postponement of death (from a specific cause) and treatment of non-fatal illnesses. The conclusions drawn in respect of non-fatal illnesses are not essentially different from those for fatal conditions: that while symptomatic relief can be provided for some, perhaps all patients, with some notable exceptions the underlying conditions cannot at present be cured.

Part Three discusses the implications of these conclusions for medicine. In relation to non-personal health services (Chapter 9) there are two important issues. One concerns public action required in the light of recognition of the significance of behavioural and environmental determinants of health; the other is related to the extent of medical involvement. Many people would say that such matters can safely be left in the hands of other health workers, a view that has attractions for some doctors who would be glad to be rid of responsibility, particularly for non-personal services. However, it is argued that a contribution is needed from medical specialists in environmental medicine and from all practising doctors in relation to patients' behaviour which prejudices their health.

Chapter 10 considers some aspects of clinical services that are related to the determinants of health. From an analysis of the tasks of clinical medicine I conclude that restoration of a 'normal' duration of life of the sick is an important goal which deserves to rank at least equally with improvement in quality of life. The design of health services is based on the assumption that investigation and treatment of disease are critical not only to recovery from acute illness, but also to long-term health prospects. It is this belief which is thought to justify the large investment in acute services, and to excuse the relative neglect of other patients, the majority, among the mentally ill, the aged sick, and the mentally subnormal. In the light of the appraisal of influences on health what is needed is not merely a transfer of resources from acute to other services, but a rethinking of the whole relationship between the various phases of care. It will also be necessary to have a more critical approach to the quality of care, including under this term: standards (how well we do what we do); effectiveness (whether what we do is worth doing); and efficiency (whether what we do makes better use of health resources than the available alternatives). Finally Chapter 10 has something to say about the relation of doctors to other health workers, already a vexed question in some fields and one that is likely to arise in others.

The implications of the conclusions from Parts One and Two for medical education are considered in Chapter 11. A health service can be no more enlightened than the minds of those who provide it, and if medical responsibilities are to be enlarged it is essential to have appropriate changes in the education of the doctor. A greater emphasis is needed on the origins of disease, the effectiveness and risks of treatment, and the care of patients who have completed investigation and treatment or who are of a kind not often seen in teaching hospitals. However, the main influence on students is undoubtedly the range of service and research interests exhibited at the teaching centre.

The direction of medical research has been determined by the belief that improvement in health depends essentially on knowledge of the body and its diseases, applied mainly through personal medical intervention in the form of immunization and therapy. In Chapter 12 it is shown that this interpretation is not in accord with past experience: the modern improvement in health was initiated and carried quite a long way with little assistance from science and technology, and until the twentieth century the contribution of science was essentially of a non-personal kind, particularly in relation to agriculture and control of water and food. However, health problems have changed in advanced countries, and the most fundamental issue confronting medical research is to evaluate two approaches to the control of disease: the first through understanding of disease mechanisms, and the second, through knowledge of disease origins. The scope for each approach is examined by placing diseases in four classes: relatively intractable; preventable, associated with poverty; preventable, associated with affluence; and potentially preventable, not known to be related to poverty or affluence.

The last two chapters bring together some general reflections on the role of medicine. Chapter 13 examines some sharply contrasted ideas which are much discussed at the present time: that residual health problems will be solved by extension of the traditional research and service methods, and the amendment: that the dream of advance through knowledge acquired in the laboratory and applied at the bedside has faded, and little more can be expected from this approach; that the goal of improved health is largely illusory, since with changing conditions of life, health problems must be expected to change but not to disappear; and that the role of medicine is essentially sinister: for many reasons, but particularly because it usurps the right of the individual to face and deal with his own health problems. Finally in Chapter 14 an attempt is made to outline the medical role in terms which take account of the nature of the residual health problems, and of the contribution which medicine can be expected to make to their solution.

2

Inheritance, Environment and Disease

When I began medical training at a London teaching hospital just before the Second World War, some observant clinicians were already aware that cancer of the lung was becoming a common disease. The surgeon who specialized in thoracic work referred frequently to the seriousness of the problem, and urged that 'Doctors must become cancer of the lung conscious, in the same way that they are already cancer of the bowel conscious.' We were told that the condition was being discovered too late for surgery to be effective, and the solution, it was implied, was in early diagnosis. So far as I can recall, there was little discussion of aetiology or of the possibility that the disease might be due to influences which could be modified or removed.

This approach to the most remarkable epidemic of the twentieth century was characteristic of the approach to disease in general. There was usually a brief comment on aetiology. (We were taught that there were five theories of toxaemia of pregnancy: if the student mentioned only four, that was one too few, and if six, one too many.) However, the discussion was mainly in mechanistic terms; in hypertension, for example, it was concerned with experimental evidence that restriction of the blood supply to the kidney raises pressure, rather than with the distribution of arterial pressure in the general population or the reasons why natural selection has failed to eliminate a serious and common disease. The focus of interest was on pathology, diagnosis, and treatment, and in the case of treatment, on what was done rather than whether it was worth doing. If clinical teachers had been asked why patients have diseases such as diabetes, hypertension, and rheumatoid arthritis, most would have discussed insulin, renal function, and allergy. And if pressed to go further and say why the underlying abnormalities exist, they would probably have referred rather vaguely to constitution, by which they would have meant inherited constitution. Infectious diseases, it would have been agreed, were essentially of environmental origin; but others, including particularly the common diseases of middle and late life, were considered to be inborn. The patient had diabetes because he had a defective pancreas and, if the matter were taken further, which usually it was not, the pancreatic abnormality was attributable to his genes.

Today the discussion of aetiology is somewhat extended, and many teachers give due attention to the importance of smoking, exercise, and diet. Moreover these influences are no longer considered only in the academic terms of a generation earlier; by their teaching and example some conscientious clinicians try to modify the practice of their students and the behaviour of their patients. Nevertheless in medicine as a whole the traditional mechanistic approach remains essentially unchanged; and it will remain unchanged so long as the concept of disease is based on a physico-chemical model.

CLASSIFICATION OF DISEASE

Textbooks of medicine rarely include a full discussion of the origin and nature of disease processes. One well-known text[1] has sections on 'genetic principles', and 'environmental factors in disease'; but these themes are considered separately, and the section on the environment is concerned mainly with topics such as heat and cold, pollution and poisoning, rather than with the relation between heredity and environment in the causation of disease.

This subject is discussed in the genetic section which is included in some, but by no means all, textbooks of medicine. Geneticists have of course written perceptively about the basis of disease, and some have examined the feasibility of control in the light of the conclusions (for example, whether familial concentration of a disease implies that it is unlikely to be influenced by environmental measures). In general, however, and understandably, they have approached the subject against the background of genetic interest, and diseases are usually divided into three classes: uncommon conditions associated with single genes; conditions (common at conception and uncommon at birth) associated with chromosomal aberrations; and common diseases whose genetic basis is obscure.

1. Cecil, R. F., and Loeb, R. F., in Beeson, P. B., and McDermott, W. (eds), *Textbook of Medicine* (Philadelphia, London, Toronto: W. B. Saunders Company, 1971), pp. 4, 24.

However, if the approach to aetiology is an operational one whose aim is prevention or some other means of control, an alternative distinction can be made between diseases according to whether they are or are not determined at fertilization. For serious conditions determined irreversibly at fertilization, the only complete solutions would be avoidance of conception or elimination during pregnancy by abortion. In contrast, diseases not established at fertilization could in principle be prevented if it were possible to identify and modify adverse environmental influences.

DISEASES DETERMINED AT FERTILIZATION

There are three types of diseases in this class, distinguishable according to whether the genetic abnormality can be seen, predicted, or inferred.

Chromosomal aberrations. Chromosomal aberrations can be seen under the microscope, and current estimates suggest that at the beginning of pregnancy they are present in about 5 per cent of embryos. Having regard to the complexity of events at fertilization, it is perhaps surprising that they are not more common. The large majority are eliminated by abortion (more than a third of spontaneous abortions appear to have abnormal chromosomes), so that their incidence in live births is low.

Single-gene disorders. These are the simply inherited abnormalities, dominant, recessive, or X-linked, whose distribution can be predicted on Mendelian principles. Where the fertility of those affected is low or absent, the frequency of the genes is reduced by natural selection, and the continued appearance of conditions such as haemophilia is attributed to new mutations. Phenylketonuria and a few similar conditions can now be treated with some success, and in time, no doubt, it will be possible to treat effectively some other single gene disorders. In this case the effects of the abnormalities would no longer be determined irreversibly at fertilization, and in an operational classification they could be transferred to conditions which can be prevented or corrected by environmental measures (which in this context include treatment).

Other abnormalities determined at fertilization. Genetic disorders which are simply inherited or due to chromosomal aberrations are observed in about 0.5 per cent of births; in classifications of disease the rest, the large majority, are usually considered together as common diseases which are polygenic. This classification brings under the common diseases some which are determined at fertilization. They are not associated with detectable abnormalities of single genes or chromosomes, and their inevitability from the time of fertilization can only be inferred. I refer particularly to certain diseases and disabilities of late life.

This interpretation rests on a conclusion which would hardly be disputed, that the maximum duration of life of a species is genetically determined. Of course it may be shortened by environmental accidents of many kinds; but it cannot be prolonged significantly beyond the normal span. Examples of exceptionally long lives of more than a hundred years are sometimes cited as evidence that life-expectancy could be increased by internal or external measures; they prove only that like other characters such as stature and intelligence, the 'natural' duration of life is distributed over a wide range. With such characters the range could be modified by selective breeding if society were prepared to accept a single major objective and to introduce stringent control of reproduction in order to achieve it. Neither possibility seems desirable or likely.

If the maximum duration of life is determined at the time of fertilization, so too, it seems reasonable to believe, are some of the diseases and disabilities associated with its end. There are mystics and others who appear to find suffering rewarding; but if allowed to choose, most people would probably elect to die in late life during sleep from a myocardial infarction or cerebral haemorrhage, the Almighty's approximation to the clinical efficiency of the abattoir. Unfortunately the execution is frequently bungled, so that the programmed end is preceded by a period of ill-health, caused by the breakdown of non-essential organs, such as eyes, ears, or joints, or by the partial collapse of an essential one, such as the brain, the heart, or the kidney, usually from a vascular accident or deficiency.

However, it is safer to conclude that some disorders of late life are genetic than to specify the ones that are. It is not long since most of the ill-named degenerative diseases would have been labelled *en bloc* as inborn, or constitutional; indeed, in his inaugural address at University College ('An Unsolved Problem of Biology') Medawar[2] examined the possibility that many serious conditions are genetically determined and occur in late life because they are unaffected or less affected by natural selection. However, it is now clear that cancer of the lung, chronic

2. Medawar, P. B., *The Uniqueness of the Individual* (London: Methuen & Co. Ltd, 1957), p. 44.

bronchitis, and some forms of heart disease are largely determined by the environment, and it is probable that the same is true for many other diseases, including most cancers. Nevertheless it would be unreasonably optimistic to believe that all the disorders of the elderly are of this kind, and it is quite likely that some defects of brain, vision, hearing, and locomotion (for example) are the result of a differential rate of wearing-out of organs determined by genes.

The grouping of this third class of conditions whose genetic basis is obscure, with the previous two for which there is a good deal of knowledge, may seem unsatisfactory; and so it is, if we are concerned primarily with the underlying mechanisms. But if our interest is in disease control, the most useful distinction is between conditions which could be eliminated only by contraception or abortion, and those in which there is the possibility of prevention by environmental measures. It is on these grounds that some abnormalities, particularly in late life, deserve to be included among diseases determined at fertilization.

DISEASES NOT DETERMINED AT FERTILIZATION

The large majority of diseases and disabilities are neither simply inherited nor otherwise determined irreversibly at fertilization; they are usually described as multifactorial, by which is meant that they are caused by interaction between multiple environmental and genetic influences. All common diseases that have been studied are to some extent familial, and attempts have been made to attribute them to a few specific genes, or to a single gene of low penetrance whose effects are irregularly manifested. The results are not convincing, and take us little beyond the conclusion that their genetic basis is obscure.

The questions of most practical importance in relation to these diseases are: Is it possible to assess the relative importance of heredity and environment? and Would such an assessment enable us to judge the feasibility of preventing a disease by modifying the environment?

NATURE AND NURTURE

The difficulty of assessing, and particularly of assessing numerically, the respective contributions of heredity and environment was discussed at some length by Hogben in *Nature and Nurture*.[3] He examined the results of temperature changes in two mutations of the fruit fly *Drosophila*

3. Hogben, L., *Nature and Nurture*, William Withering Memorial Lecture, 1935 (London: George Allen and Unwin Ltd, 1945), p. 96.

which differ in the number of eye facets: the number of facets varies with the temperature of the environment in which the larvae develop (Fig. 2.1). It was observed that there was a difference between the number of facets (*a*) in the two stocks at the same temperature attributable to the genetic difference (represented by AB at 16°C and EF at 25°C) and (*b*) in the same stock at different temperatures, attributable to the environmental difference (for the change of temperature

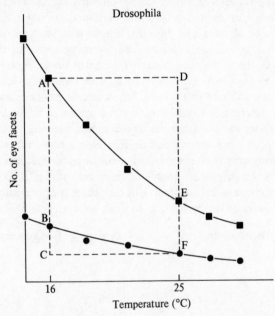

FIGURE 2.1. Number of eye facets in two mutations of *Drosophila* according to the temperature of the environment in which the larvae develop.

Source: L. Hogben, *Nature and Nurture*, George Allen and Unwin Ltd. 1945, p. 96.

from 16°C to 25°C, represented by DE for one and by BC for the other). But it was not possible to assess the contributions of heredity and environment when comparing the number of facets in the two stocks in different environments. Hogben concluded: 'We are on safe ground when we speak of genetic difference between two groups measured in one and the same environment or in speaking of a difference due to the environment when identical stocks are measured under different

conditions of development.' But we are not on equally safe ground
when we speak of the contribution of heredity and environment to
the measurements of genetically different individuals measured in different kinds of environment.

The conclusions from the observations on *Drosophila* may be ampli-
fied by reference to a human disease. Let us consider two individuals
who differ in their genetically determined proneness to diabetes. In rural
Africa, on the traditional diet, neither would exhibit the disease; in a
western country, on refined foods with a high intake of sugar, the more
prone might be affected and the other might not. We can conclude
that the difference in the experience of the more prone in the two
countries was due to the change in diet, and that the difference in the
disease experience of the two individuals in the western country was
probably attributable to their genes. But comparing the experience of
the two in different environments, we can arrive at no meaningful
conclusion about the contributions of nature and nurture.

The interplay of inheritance and environment across a range of different environments is illustrated further in the models shown in Fig.
2.2. The first compares the response of three pure strains (A, B and C)
to changes in the environment; in this case there is no variation, and
the differences (large between A and B, small between B and C) are due

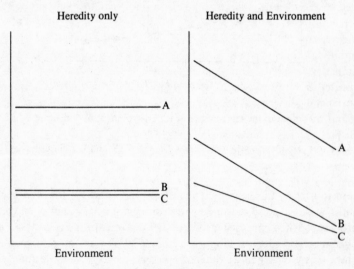

FIGURE 2.2. Model illustrating the interaction of heredity and
environment.

to heredity only. The second model compares strains whose responses vary in relation to both heredity and environment; but the difference between A and B remains constant over the environmental range whereas that between B and C (and A and C) varies.

Although these models are theoretical, they undoubtedly illustrate some of the problems of interpretation of the influence of heredity and environment in the aetiology of disease. Diseases determined at fertilization are represented by the first model, in the sense that their manifestation is independent of the environment. However, most abnormalities, including the common diseases, are not of this kind. They are due to the interaction of genetic and environmental influences, whose relative contributions vary between diseases and for the same disease in different environments.

In the light of these difficulties we need to be extremely cautious when attempting to assess, particularly in quantitative terms, the effects of heredity and environment in the causation of human disease. There are no pure strains and there are few constant environments; conclusions must therefore be based on investigations which are no more than approximations to the experimental models.

The only individuals with identical genes are monozygotic twins, and observed differences in their disease experience can usually be attributed to their environments, prenatal or post-natal. (Even about this conclusion there must be a reservation: Edwards has noted that 'differences between similar cells in similar tissues must be largely fortuitous and it would be wrong to infer that, because identical twins show little similarity in their liability to some diseases, particularly such focal diseases as neoplasia, environmental features must, therefore, be important'.)[4] However, the matter is usually considered the other way round: if identical twins are consistently both affected in different environments, the abnormality is said to be determined by their common genes. The usual procedure is to identify pairs in which at least one twin is affected, and inquire how frequently the other twin has the same condition (ie, is concordant). The results are then compared with those of dizygotic twins and, sometimes, other relatives. In no common disease is concordance 100 per cent; but when it is consistently high in twins exposed to different environments, say over 80 per cent and at least twice the rate in non-identical twins, it seems permissible to conclude that the condition is largely determined by genes of high specificity.

4. Edwards, J. H., 'The genetic basis of common disease', *American Journal of Medicine*, **34** (1963), p. 631.

In practice it is of course difficult to find a considerable number of identical twins with a disorder, even a common one, who have been observed in different environments. It must also be remembered that twins are unusual in both their intra-uterine environment and their upbringing, so there must be reservations when generalizing from experience of twins to that of single births.

The second possibility is to examine the disease experience of individuals who differ genetically but share the same environment. The usual method is to compare identical twins whose genes are common, with other relatives (parents, children, sibs) in whom half the genes are the same. Different genotypes are also identifiable by blood groups and, less reliably, by markers such as race and colour. The general problem with this approach is uncertainty that the environments to which those compared have been exposed were the same, at least in respect of the features, often unknown, which are critical for the disease in question. Since close relatives share a common environment as well as common genes, it is hardly surprising that many diseases tend to run in families and from this observation alone no conclusion can be drawn about the contributions of heredity and environment.

The problem in applying the two approaches to the study of human disease is not therefore that they are wrong in principle, but that in practice it is often impossible to assemble the requisite data. It is difficult to find a large number of affected individuals of the same genotype (identical twins) exposed to a range of different environments, or of different genotypes exposed to the same environment. What is usually available is a comparison between different genotypes observed in different environments, and the interpretation is open to the objections referred to above.

In spite of these difficulties it is possible to arrive at tentative conclusions about the contribution of heredity and environment in some diseases. For example, nearly everyone who eats food infected by salmonella organisms suffers from gastro-enteritis, but only a small proportion of those exposed to respiratory tuberculosis contract the clinical disease. (On the latter point perhaps the best evidence is the low frequency of tuberculosis in wives of men who are sputum positive.) In the one case the salmonella organisms are a necessary and (almost) a sufficient condition for the appearance of the disease in man; in the other the tubercle bacillus is a necessary but not a sufficient condition, since it requires the complement of the appropriate genotype. But does this distinction have much bearing on the feasibility of control?

FEASIBILITY OF CONTROL

This brings us to the second question concerning the common diseases: Does assessment of the contribution of nature and nurture enable us to judge the possibility of preventing a disease by modifying the environment?

In the case of infectious diseases the answer turns to a considerable extent on the ways they are spread. It is relatively easy to interrupt transmission of water-borne diseases (such as cholera and typhoid) by control of the public supply; it is more difficult to prevent the spread of food-borne diseases (such as salmonella and staphylococcal poisoning) which requires strict personal hygiene; and it is often impossible to control airborne infections (such as pneumonia, influenza, and the common cold).

With non-communicable diseases the problems are much greater, and for a number of reasons. The nature of the adverse influences may be unknown, as in schizophrenia and breast cancer; they may be multiple, and hence difficult to assess, as in coronary artery disease; or their removal may require modification of behaviour which many people are reluctant to accept, as in cancer of the lung and road accidents. But by far the most important restriction exists where the influences are prenatal, and difficult or impossible to identify or control. Indeed, in relation to the feasibility of prevention, the distinction between congenital conditions and those determined after birth is more important than that between infections and non-communicable diseases; it is also more significant than the balance sheet of heredity and environment.

This appraisal of heredity and environment in the aetiology of disease suggests that improvement in health is likely to result from elimination of environmental hazards, and to be in respect of conditions determined post-natally rather than prenatally. This conclusion is consistent with the age-trend of mortality in England and Wales between 1838–54 and 1970. Fig. 2.3 shows the number of deaths per 1,000 conceptions for five age periods: prenatal, 0–14, 15–44, 45–64, and 65 and over. Mortality after birth was estimated by applying to the numbers live-born (estimated as 770 per 1,000 conceptions in both 1838–54 and 1970) data provided in English life tables for the relevant years. The only uncertainties are about prenatal losses, which are based on the figures in Table 2.1.

Contemporary estimates of the proportions of conceptions aborted spontaneously appear to be reasonably reliable and are about 140 per

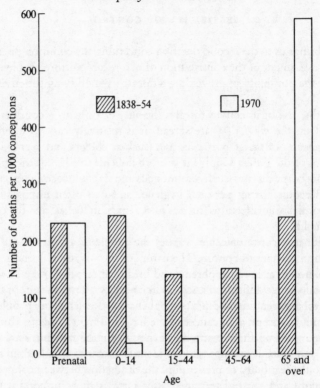

FIGURE 2.3. Mortality at different ages: England and Wales.

1,000; there is no reason to believe that this figure has changed greatly since the mid nineteenth century. The frequency of legal abortions has risen rapidly since the liberalization of the grounds for abortion in 1968 and the figure for 1970 (70 per 1,000) is based on the number of legal abortions reported for that year.

Estimates of illegal abortions are the least reliable, and even today their number is unknown. But since the change in the law the number of pregnancies terminated illegally is probably small, and it has been assumed to be 10 per 1,000. The figure for 1838–54 (50 per 1,000) can be no more than a guess. On the one hand it seems certain that it was higher than it is today; on the other hand the methods available for inducing abortion were restricted and unwanted children were sometimes eliminated by infanticide.

The estimate for stillbirths in 1970 is based on the stillbirth rate

TABLE 2.1. *Estimates of prenatal deaths in 1838–54 and 1970: England and Wales*

	Deaths per 1,000 conceptions	
	1838–54	1970
Spontaneous abortions	140	140
Legal abortions	Nil	70
Illegal abortions	50	10
Stillbirths	40	10
Total	230	230

(number of stillbirths per 1,000 stillbirths and live-births) for that year. For 1838–54, when stillbirths were not recorded, the rate has been assumed to be 50; the earliest recorded rate was 40 in 1928. This gives an estimate of approximately 40 stillbirths per 1,000 conceptions when account is taken of abortions.

On these estimates, the proportion of conceptions which terminate prenatally is of the order of 20 to 25 per cent. So far as can be judged from the limited data, the proportion has not altered substantially since the mid nineteenth century.

Fig. 2.3 shows the remarkable change in the distribution of deaths during the past century. The notable features are: (*a*) little change in prenatal deaths (in spite of the decline of the stillbirth rate, whose contribution to the total of prenatal losses is not large); (*b*) a reduction in the number of deaths in early and middle life, marked at ages 0–14 and 15–44 and small at 45–64; and (*c*) an increase in deaths at 65 and over. This increase is of course due mainly to the greater number of people surviving to late life.

These trends in the age distribution of mortality are in accord with the interpretation outlined above. Prenatal mortality remains high, not because the causes of death are determined mainly at fertilization (although some, particularly the chromosomal aberrations, undoubtedly are), but because the hazards associated with implantation and early embryonic development are largely unidentified. The great reduction of deaths in early life was due to environmental measures which reduced the prevalence and case-fatality of the predominant infections. But has there also been a substantial reduction of mortality at later ages, which is masked in Fig. 2.3 by the increased numbers surviving to late life?

National estimates indicate that there has been some increase in life expectation, say at ages 45 and over, but it has been much smaller than at younger ages. This might be interpreted to mean that the so-called degenerative diseases cannot be expected to decline because they are determined at the time of fertilization and, being in the post-reproductive age period, are removed from the effects of natural selection.

A few decades ago it would have been difficult to reject this conclusion. However, it is now clear that some of the common causes of death in middle and late life are largely determined by the environment; for example, chronic bronchitis and coronary artery disease. But perhaps the most impressive grounds for believing that many deaths in this age period are preventable is the evidence that most cancers are due to influences which in principle could be modified.[5]

Against this background it can be said that while infections differ from other common diseases in the case of their control, they do not differ in the concept of their origin. In both cases a certain genotype is needed, but its ill-effects are manifested only in a suitable environment. In practice the important consideration is not the balance sheet of nature and nurture (assuming that it could be quantified) but the feasibility of identifying and removing the adverse influences. This conclusion is consistent with recognition that some disorders, mainly of late life, are genetically determined, in the sense that, like the duration of life, they are programmed at the time of fertilization.

I shall now attempt to summarize conclusions which follow from this appraisal of heredity and environment in relation to human diseases, and to consider briefly the implications for the means of their control. Diseases and disabilities can be divided broadly into four classes as follows.

CONDITIONS DETERMINED AT FERTILIZATION

(a) *Genetic diseases*. This term is interpreted to include both single gene disorders, which are simply inherited, and chromosomal aberrations which are largely eliminated as abortions. Genetic diseases, so defined, are uncommon among abnormalities manifested at birth or in post-natal life.

(b) *Other diseases determined at fertilization*. These comprise mainly conditions associated with the genetically programmed wearing-out

5. Doll, R., *Prevention of Cancer. Pointers from Epidemiology*. Rock Carling Monograph (Nuffield Provincial Hospitals Trust, 1967), p. 129.

of organs at the end of life. They are not simply inherited, but are attributable to multiple genes which are nevertheless highly specific.

CONDITIONS WHICH OCCUR ONLY IN AN APPROPRIATE ENVIRONMENT

(c) *Diseases in which the environmental influences are prenatal.* These include most abortions and stillbirths, congenital abnormalities (such as malformations and most cases of mental subnormality) and some conditions which first come to attention in post-natal life (most non-infective disorders of childhood are determined by the time of birth). These diseases are attributable to unknown influences within the uterus operating on genetic material whose character is also obscure.

(d) *Diseases in which the environmental influences are post-natal.* They comprise conditions, both infective and non-infective, which, so far as is known, are not due to influences before birth. They probably include nearly all the common diseases and disabilities (accidents, diabetes, peptic ulcer, rheumatoid arthritis, psychiatric disorders, etc.) as well as others such as the cancers which formerly would have been attributed to inborn constitution (class (b) above). They are usually described as multifactorial, which tells us little more than that their aetiology is complex and their genetic basis obscure.

I shall examine the implications of this classification more closely in Chapters 7 and 12 but three comments should be made at this point. One is that diseases in the first three classes are all relatively intractable, but for quite different reasons: the first two because they are determined at fertilization, and the third because environmental influences during pregnancy are difficult to recognize and control. Second, the age trend of mortality in the past century is what would be expected from the classification: little improvement before birth and a large reduction post-natally, mainly in younger age-groups, brought about by a decline of deaths from diseases in the fourth class. And third, in principle all the diseases in the fourth class could be prevented by appropriate environmental modifications; but in practice control of infections is often relatively simple, whereas control of non-communicable diseases may be difficult or impossible.

Part Two
Determinants of Health

3

Decline of Mortality

Although the documentary evidence was very unsatisfactory before births and deaths were registered nationally, there is no doubt that there has been a vast improvement in health during the last three centuries. During most of man's existence it is probable that a considerable proportion of all children died or were killed within a few years of birth. Such records as are available, taken with recent experience in developing countries, suggest that although there was considerable variation from time to time and from place to place, out of 10 newborn children, on average, 2–3 died before the first birthday, 5–6 by age 6 and about 7 before maturity. In technologically advanced countries today, more than 95 per cent survive to adult life.

The decline of mortality, and the associated increase in expectation of life at birth – from between 30 and 40 years in 1700 to 72 years for males and 77 for females in the country (Sweden) with the best figures in 1970 – are not the only indications of improvement in health. Still less are they a sufficient basis for discussion of the medical role, and Chapter 8 examines other indices of medical achievement; the postponement of death and treatment of morbidity from diseases which do not kill. Nevertheless, it will be suggested that if priority is to be given among measures which are all desirable, the prevention of death and extension of life were the most important achievements. It is therefore essential to determine the reasons for the decline of mortality.

The earliest national records of births and deaths are for Sweden (from 1751) and France (from 1800) and they leave no doubt that death-rates were falling from the beginning of the nineteenth century. However, there is impressive indirect evidence that the decline began somewhat earlier, probably in the first half of the eighteenth century, in the rapid growth of population which was evident in many countries before 1800. Attempts have been made to attribute this expansion largely to a rise in birth-rates, brought about by withdrawal of

29

restraints on fertility. This explanation is not convincing, since it can readily be shown that if mortality had not declined the populations would not have risen. Any increase from rising birth-rates in the eighteenth century would have been offset by their subsequent fall from the nineteenth century.[1].

When interpreting the decline of mortality we must rely to a considerable extent on what is admittedly an unreliable source of evidence, namely, national statistics of cause of death. However, in spite of their deficiencies (discussed below) these data are of considerable value. They were available first in England and Wales (from 1838). In the years immediately after registration the records were incomplete or for other reasons unsatisfactory, but from 1841 it is possible to examine the trend of mortality associated with specific diseases. This evidence from national sources from the first half of the nineteenth century is not available elsewhere, so in other countries interpretation is virtually restricted to the twentieth century. This may explain the frequent over-estimation of the contribution of immunization and therapy, since these measures have had their impact mainly, indeed with one exception (vaccination against smallpox) probably wholly, since 1900.

THE TREND OF MORTALITY

Fig. 3.1 shows the death-rate for males and females from 1841 to 1971. For the nineteenth century the rates are for the six decades and for the twentieth century they are for the first year of each decade; both were standardized in relation to the 1901 population to correct for the changing age structure, since with an ageing population the crude death-rates underestimate the reduction of mortality which actually occured. Throughout the period death-rates were considerably higher for males than for females; they began to fall in the eighth decade of the nineteenth century and the decline has continued to the present day.

However, as already noted, the examination cannot be restricted to the nineteenth and twentieth centuries, since the growth of population (in England and Wales it trebled between 1700 and 1851) indicates that the decline of the death-rate began well before 1838. Table 3.1 shows the proportion of the reduction of mortality which occurred in three periods: 1700 to the mid nineteenth century (a third); the second half

1. McKeown, T. 'Fertility, mortality and causes of death', *Population Studies*, 32 (1978), p. 535.

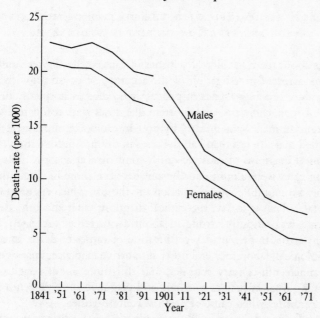

FIGURE 3.1. Death-rates (standardized to 1901 population):
England and Wales.

of the nineteenth century (a fifth); and the twentieth century (nearly
half). These figures are based on the assumption that the death-rate in
England and Wales at the beginning of the eighteenth century was 30.
The Swedish death-rate for the period 1751 to 1800 was 27.4 and the
rate for England and Wales is believed to have been at about the same
level or a little higher.

TABLE 3.1. *Reduction of mortality since 1700: England and Wales*

Period	Percentage of total reduction in each period*	Percentage of reduction due to infections
1700 to 1848–54	33	?
1848–54 to 1901	20	92
1901 to 1971	47	73
1700 to 1971	100	

*The estimates are based on the assumption that the death-rate in 1700 was 30.

DISEASES ASSOCIATED WITH THE DECLINE OF MORTALITY
AFTER REGISTRATION OF BIRTHS AND DEATHS

Doubts about the reliability of statistics of cause of death were under-
lined by a recent investigation of the accuracy of certification in the
present day. In a large series of patients who died in hospitals during
1975 and 1976, clinicians' ante-mortem diagnoses were compared with
the diagnoses made subsequently by post-mortem examination. It was
concluded that: 'In less than half the cases in this prospective study was
the clinical diagnosis of cause of death confirmed at autopsy. The remaining cases were almost equally split between those in which there
was only a minor difference of opinion and those in which disagreement
was total.'[2] That is to say, the clinical diagnosis entered on the death
certificate was seriously wrong in about a quarter of the cases. The
frequent errors in present-day certification of causes of death, in spite
of radiological, laboratory and other supportive evidence, raise doubts
about nineteenth-century statistics, and still more about conclusions
concerning diseases such as smallpox and plague in the eighteenth and
earlier centuries when cause of death was not certified.

The difficulties are particularly serious in diseases such as pneumonia,
where the evidence is prejudiced not only by errors in diagnosis but
also by changes in diagnostic fashions and in classification of cause of
death. Scarlet fever, for example, was not separated from diphtheria
in the national classification in England and Wales until 1855, nor typhus
from typhoid until 1869. It is therefore important to consider some of
the main questions in relation to the infections as a whole, or at least in
relation to broad classes (such as airborne or water- and food-borne
diseases), rather than to put too much weight on interpretation of the
behaviour of any single disease. Nevertheless, something can be learned
from an examination of single diseases, if their special features and the
considerable range of error within which the statistics are likely to fall
are taken into account.

In the discussion which follows conditions attributable to micro-
organisms are distinguished from conditions which are not. The
distinction cannot be made in all cases. For example, in the early registration period rheumatic heart disease was not separated from other
diseases of the heart, so although caused by streptococcal infection, it
is included with non-infective conditions. Nephritis was classified with

2. Waldron, H. A. and Vickerstaff, L., *Intimations of Quality. Ante-mortem and
post-mortem diagnoses* (London: Nuffield Provincial Hospitals Trust, 1977).

dropsy which is partly of non-infective origin, so when data for the mid nineteenth century are used nephritis is also taken with conditions not attributable to micro-organisms, although most cases result from infection. There are a few other infective conditions which even today cannot be separated in national statistics, for example diseases of the heart and nervous system due to syphilis and congenital malformations which result from rubella. With these reservations, the broad distinction between infective and non-infective conditions can be made with reasonable confidence

Table 3.1 shows the proportion of the decline of mortality associated with infectious diseases, 92 per cent from 1848–54 to 1901 and 73 per cent from 1901 to 1971. On the assumption that there was no decrease in non-infective deaths before 1838 when cause of death was unknown, 86 per cent of the total reduction of the death-rate from the beginning of the eighteenth century to the present day was attributable to the decline of the infections.

INFECTIONS

In Table 3.2 the reduction of mortality associated with infectious diseases is divided between three groups: airborne; water-and food-borne; and other. The years 1848–54 have been taken to represent the beginning of the registration period because certification of cause of death

TABLE 3.2. *Reduction of mortality, 1848–54 to 1971:*
England and Wales

	Percentage of reduction
Conditions attributable to micro-organisms	
1. Airborne diseases	40
2. Water- and food-borne diseases	21
3. Other conditions	13
Total	74
Conditions not attributable to micro-organisms	26
All diseases	100

The estimate of the proportion of deaths associated with micro-organisms is lower than would be suggested by Table 3.1, because when the whole period (1848–54 to 1971) is considered, certain infections (for example rheumatic fever) cannot be included.

was incomplete during part of the first decade after registration, and the rates for 1848–54 and 1971 were standardized to correspond with the age distribution of the 1901 population. Of the fall of mortality since the mid nineteenth century, 40 per cent was from airborne diseases, 21 per cent from water- and food-borne diseases, 13 per cent from other infections, and the remainder (26 per cent) from non-infective conditions.

Airborne diseases. Table 3.3 shows the contribution made by different airborne diseases to the total decline of mortality. Respiratory tuberculosis accounted for 17.5 per cent, and more than half of this improvement occurred before the end of the nineteenth century. Mortality from the disease fell continuously, at least from the time when cause of death was first registered, and by the fifth decade it had fallen by about a quarter.

TABLE 3.3. *Standardized death-rates (per million) from airborne diseases: England and Wales*

	1848–54	1971	Percentage of reduction from all causes attributable to each disease
Tuberculosis (respiratory)	2,901	13	17.5
Bronchitis, pneumonia, influenza	2,239	603	9.9
Whooping cough	423	1	2.6
Measles	342	0	2.1
Scarlet fever and diphtheria	1,016	0	6.2
Smallpox	263	0	1.6
Infections of ear, pharynx, larynx	75	2	0.4
Total	7,259	619	40.3

The next largest contribution was from bronchitis, pneumonia, (as in Table 3.3) influenza (9.9 per cent). It is unfortunately necessary to group these conditions because there is some evidence of transfers from one to another. For example, both pneumonia and bronchitis deaths show an increase in years of high influenza prevalence, and it seems clear that a number of influenza deaths were ascribed to pneumonia, and, even more frequently, to bronchitis. Confusion between bronchitis and pneumonia, at least in old people, is suggested by the fact that the death-rate of men aged 75 and over attributed to pneumonia increased between 1901 and 1971, whereas deaths from bronchitis decreased. It is also possible that some deaths which earlier would have been certified as 'old age' were transferred to this category, in which case the number of deaths from these respiratory diseases would have been larger in 1901 and the decline by 1971 correspondingly greater. The trend of mortality will be examined more closely later, but here it should be noted that there is evidence that the reduction of the death-rate from pneumonia, bronchitis, and influenza began before the end of the nineteenth century.

Diphtheria and scarlet fever were associated with 6.2 per cent of the fall of mortality and three-fifths of the decline occurred before 1901. The diseases can be separated after 1855; the death-rate from scarlet fever fell rapidly in the second half of the nineteenth century, whereas that from diphtheria increased slightly. Since 1901 both have declined, and there have been few deaths from either disease in England and Wales since 1951.

Whooping cough contributed 2.6 per cent to the reduction of mortality. The decrease was relatively small in the nineteenth century and accounted for only about a quarter of the fall between 1848–54 and 1971. Nevertheless mortality from the disease has declined almost continuously since about 1870, and there are now few deaths in England and Wales (26 in 1971, of which 22 were in children under 1 year).

Measles was associated with 2.1 per cent of the fall of the death-rate. During the nineteenth and early twentieth centuries childhood mortality from measles was relatively high, but it fell rapidly from about the time of the First World War. Nevertheless measles remains an important disease; in 1971, 135,000 cases were notified and there were 28 deaths.

Smallpox contributed 1.6 per cent to the reduction of the death-rate and almost all of this improvement occurred before 1901. Since about 1910 there have been few deaths from smallpox in the British Isles.

It seems unnecessary to comment in detail on the remaining infections (of ear, pharynx, and larynx), which accounted for only 0.4 per cent of the fall of mortality. There are also some airborne diseases which caused few deaths and have been classified under 'other conditions'.

Water- and food-borne diseases. Water- and food-borne diseases (Table 3.4) were associated with about a fifth of the fall of the death-rate between 1848–54 and 1971; nearly half of the improvement occurred before 1901.

TABLE 3.4. *Standardized death-rates (per million) from water- and food-borne diseases: England and Wales*

	1848–54	1971	Percentage of reduction from all causes attributable to each disease
Cholera, diarrhoea, dysentery	1,819	33	10.8
Tuberculosis (non-respiratory)	753	2	4.6
Typhoid, typhus	990	0	6.0
Total	3,562	35	21.4

It seems desirable to group together the diarrhoeal diseases. In the twentieth century they comprised essentially diarrhoea, dysentery, and enteritis; but in the period 1848–54 there were also a considerable number of deaths attributed to cholera which are included under the same heading. These diseases were responsible for about a tenth of the fall in mortality before 1971; a third of the decline occurred before 1901.

Deaths associated with non-respiratory tuberculosis in 1848–54 are those shown in the Registrar-General's classification as scrofula, *tabes mesenteri*, and hydrocephalus. Deaths attributed to hydrocephalus include some due to the congenital and other forms of the disease; however, in the nineteenth century most deaths were undoubtedly from tuberculous meningitis, and since the different types were not then separated in national statistics, it seems right to classify them with other forms of non-respiratory tuberculosis. This overstatement of non-respiratory tuberculosis deaths is offset by the inevitable omission of deaths due to renal and bone and joint tuberculosis. From 1901 the classification was reasonably comprehensive, and there is little difficulty in following the trend of mortality from that time. The disease was responsible for 4.6 per cent of the reduction of the death-rate between 1848–54 and 1971 and about a quarter of the improvement occurred before 1901.

Since typhus was not distinguished from typhoid fever before 1869, they are considered together in Table 3.4. It is unfortunate that this grouping is necessary, since typhus is not spread by water and food and should be included under 'other conditions'. The balance of deaths due to typhus and typhoid before 1869 is uncertain, but from that time at least the latter greatly outnumbered the former. The death-rate from typhus fell rapidly in the last decade of the nineteenth century and there have been few deaths during the twentieth. Together these diseases were associated with 6 per cent of the reduction of mortality between 1848–54 and 1971, of which 84 per cent occurred before 1901.

It should be noted that the rate of decline of mortality before the turn of the century was much greater for the enteric diseases, spread mainly by water, than for the diarrhoeal diseases spread mainly by food.

Other diseases due to micro-organisms. There remains a miscellaneous group of conditions of infective origin, which are not spread mainly by air, water, or food, or for which certification of cause of death was unsatisfactory (as in the case of 'convulsions and teething'). Diseases of this class were responsible for 12.6 per cent of the fall of mortality between 1848–54 and 1971 and about a third of this decrease occurred before 1901.

Table 3.5 shows the contribution made by different conditions; the largest (8 per cent) was from 'convulsions and teething'. Although these terms were long regarded as unsatisfactory, they were still employed in 1901 when 20,956 deaths were attributed to them. By 1911 the term

TABLE 3.5. *Standardized death-rates (per million) for other diseases attributable to micro-organisms: England and Wales*

	1848–54	1971	Percentage of reduction from all causes attributable to each disease
Convulsions, teething	1,322	0	8.0
Syphilis	50	0	0.3
Appendicitis, peritonitis	75	7	0.4
Puerperal fever	62	1	0.4
Other infections	635	52	3.5
Total	2,144	60	12.6

teething was no longer accepted, although it was still used in association with 'convulsions'. The use of 'convulsions' also diminished; only 9 deaths were certified in 1961 and none in 1971. This decrease was presumably due mainly to transfer of deaths to other and more acceptable causes, as well as to the general decline of the underlying infections.

Most of these deaths were infective. They were associated particularly with diseases of childhood (whooping cough, measles, otitis media, meningitis, pneumonia, gastro-enteritis, etc.), and in this analysis attention has been restricted to deaths under 5 years in the Registrar-General's

reports. Although it is not possible to identify the causes of death included under convulsions and teething, it is probable that most of them
were airborne infections.

The other diseases specified in Table 3.5 contributed little to the decline of mortality: syphilis, 0.3 per cent; appendicitis and peritonitis,
0.4 per cent; and puerperal fever, 0.4 per cent. Except in the case of
appendicitis there are no special difficulties in identifying these conditions in the Registrar-General's classification. Syphilis is taken to include
the principle manifestations of the disease: general paralysis of the insane,
locomotor ataxia, and aneurysm. Until 1951 the frequency of deaths
from cardiovascular syphilis was slightly understated, because the classification did not separate those due to syphilitic valvular disease. Until
1931 the number of deaths attributed to puerperal fever was also low
because infective deaths associated with abortion were not identified.

NON-INFECTIVE CONDITIONS

The conditions under this heading (Table 3.6) are a heterogeneous
collection, having in common only that they are not due to micro-
organisms or, where they are, that they cannot be identified in
national statistics. Together these conditions were associated with 25.6
per cent of the decline of mortality since 1848–54 and a tenth of this
reduction occurred before 1901.

There are many problems of terminology and classification. For example, the term 'old age' was common, and although it was recognized
to be unsatisfactory more than a fifth of the deaths of persons aged 65
and over were attributed to it in 1901. From 1911 the use of the term
diminished, deaths presumably being transferred to more acceptable
causes, both infectious (for example pneumonia) and non-infectious
(heart disease). This category of deaths contributed 8.7 per cent to the
decline.

The heading 'prematurity, immaturity, and other diseases of infancy',
associated with 6.2 per cent of the decline, undoubtedly covers a large
number of very different conditions. As knowledge of neonatal diseases
increased, the classification was expanded, and some deaths were transferred to more satisfactory categories. However, these distinctions cannot be made in the nineteenth and early twentieth centuries, so it is
necessary to combine prematurity with other diseases of infancy. Deaths
in this class increased in the late nineteenth century, and did not decline

TABLE 3.6. *Standardized death-rates (per million) from conditions not attributable to micro-organisms: England and Wales*

	1848–54	1971	Percentage of reduction from all causes attributable to each condition
Congenital defects	28	127	0.6 increase
Prematurity, immaturity, other diseases of infancy	1,221	192	6.2
Cerebrovascular disease	890	603	1.7
Cardiovascular disease	698	1,776	6.5 increase
Cancer	307	1,169	5.2 increase
Other diseases of digestive system	706	105	3.6
Other diseases of nervous system	316	63	1.5
Nephritis	615	46	3.5
Other diseases of urinary system	107	23	0.5
Pregnancy and childbirth (excluding sepsis)	130	3	0.8
Violence	761	345	2.5
Old age	1,447	16	8.7
Other diseases	1,665	202	8.9
Total	8,891	4,670	25.6

until 1901. This largely accounts for the delay in the fall of infant mortality.

Difficulties arise with 'other diseases of the nervous system'. For example, poliomyelitis was not specified in the 1901 and 1911 classifications, and was probably grouped with 'diseases of the cord' which therefore include a few infective deaths. However, the error is small, for poliomyelitis was not then or later a common cause of death. Paralysis agitans did not appear in 1901 and 1911, but has been included since 1921 although some cases are believed to result from virus infection. This may be true also of multiple sclerosis, shown separately from 1921.

These examples, which could be extended, are characteristic of the problems of terminology and classification which arise with conditions not attributable to micro-organisms. There is a further difficulty. In the case of the infections the division according to mode of transmission will facilitate interpretation of reasons for their decline. No such approach is possible in the case of non-infective causes of death. For example, cancer mortality has increased during this century; this increase is mainly the result of deaths from lung cancer caused by smoking, and it has masked a fall of mortality from some other cancers, brought about by therapy and, no doubt, other influences. The picture is also complex in cardiovascular disease, where a large increase in deaths from myocardial infarction may have obscured a reduction from other forms. The contribution of treatment in cases of violence is probably understated because of an increase in the frequency of severe injuries.

It should be noted that the reduction of mortality was lower for males than for females (21.3 per cent and 31.6 per cent respectively in the twentieth century). This sex difference is due partly to the increase in male deaths from lung cancer and cardiovascular disease, without which the fall in male mortality from non-infectious deaths would have been much larger. This means that the decline of mortality for male non-smokers has been considerably greater than the figures suggest.

DISEASES ASSOCIATED WITH THE DECLINE OF MORTALITY BEFORE REGISTRATION

INFECTIONS

With the probable exceptions of infanticide and starvation (discussed below), the fall of mortality before registration of cause of death, as in the period from registration to 1900, was almost certainly due to a reduction of deaths from infectious diseases. As a preliminary to interpretation of the reasons for this reduction, it is desirable to consider the nature of the diseases which declined. For the pre-registration period there are no reliable data concerning individual diseases, so one must draw largely on later experience.

From 1838 the infections which declined were mainly of two types: airborne, and water- and food-borne. Mortality from some airborne infections, particularly tuberculosis, fell from the time of registration, but the decline from water- and food-borne diseases was delayed until the last decades of the nineteenth century.

It is probable that there was a substantial reduction of mortality from airborne infections in the pre-registration period. The number of deaths from tuberculosis fell rapidly from 1838, and the disease was associated with nearly half of the decrease of the death-rate during the second half of the nineteenth century. Mortality from tuberculosis was considerable in the seventeenth and eighteenth centuries, and the fact that it was declining at the time of registration suggests that it may have fallen earlier.

Another airborne infection from which deaths must have decreased before 1838 is smallpox. In 1848–54 the death-rate from the disease was only 263 (per million), less than a tenth of the rate for respiratory tuberculosis and considerably lower than the rates from whooping cough and measles (Table 3.3). We can be less confident about the trend of mortality from other airborne infections. Diphtheria was confused with scarlet fever and there is no reliable information about deaths from diseases such as whooping cough, measles, bronchitis, pneumonia, and influenza.

Evidence concerning water- and food-borne diseases is also lacking. Mortality was not falling in the decades after registration, and did not begin to decline until there were improvements in water and sewage disposal, in England and Wales from the seventh decade. Indeed the expansion of population and the rapid movement from country to towns must have increased exposure to infections spread by water and food, and the appearance of cholera, possibly for the first time, indicates that hygienic conditions deteriorated.

Finally, we must consider the possible significance of the vector-borne diseases (plague, typhus, and malaria) spread by rats, lice, and mosquitoes. These diseases were relatively unimportant after registration: plague almost disappeared from the British Isles after 1679, and although cases were introduced occasionally through seaports, no extension of the disease occurred; few deaths were attributed to typhus after 1869, when it was distinguished from typhoid; and although there may have been some indigenous cases of malaria, most deaths have resulted from infection acquired overseas.

Judged by the attention paid to it by historians, plague was the most important of the vector-borne diseases in relation to the decline of mortality and growth of population in earlier centuries. However, since the disease virtually disappeared after 1679, it cannot have been associated with the decrease of deaths from 1700.

Typhus was not differentiated from bubonic plague until about the middle of the nineteenth century and was probably responsible for many of the deaths attributed to that disease. Malaria could not be identified reliably from many other fevers before the late nineteenth century, and in the early Registrar-General's reports it was presumably included under a term such as intermittent fever. In view of the lack of evidence one can attempt only a personal appraisal. It seems probable that there were epidemics of typhus, particularly affecting the poor, at intervals during the pre-registration period, and that mortality declined until the disease virtually disappeared in the late nineteenth century. It is unlikely that malaria was ever an important cause of death in Britain; climatic conditions are not really suited to the parasite, since a temperature of not less than 20°C is required before the sexual cycle of *Plasmodium falciparum* (the cause of malignant subtertian malaria) can be completed in the mosquito, and 15°C is needed for other species.

In this assessment vector-borne diseases are assigned a much less significant place in the history of mortality than the one they occupy in developing countries today. The reason is clear. The developing countries are in or near the tropics, where climatic conditions are ideal for many parasites and animal vectors: particularly flies, mosquitoes, and snails, with the result that diseases such as dysentery, malaria, yellow fever, and schistosomiasis are endemic over large areas. But in temperate regions conditions were unsuitable for most diseases spread by animal vectors. In a sense other than they intended there is truth in the Webbs' observation that England (like most of western Europe) has the worst weather and the best climate in the world.

NON-INFECTIVE CONDITIONS

Table 3.1 suggested that in the period from 1848–54 to 1901, non-infective conditions were associated with 8 per cent of the decline of mortality. Most of this reduction was in two classes of deaths, 'old age' and 'other diseases', neither of which provides convincing evidence of a decline. The term old age was used in respect of both infections and non-infective conditions, and the fact that in this period there was a considerable increase of deaths certified as bronchitis, pneumonia and influenza, and 'other cardiovascular diseases', suggests that the apparent fall in 'old age' deaths resulted mainly from a transfer to these categories. The other diseases comprised a large and heterogeneous group of conditions, many of which were unsatisfactorily classified (for example haemorrhage, mortification, and insanity). Moreover, the reduction of deaths was mainly in two categories. One consisted of 'asthma and diseases of lungs, etc.' Many of the deaths attributed to these causes were probably associated with respiratory infections, and the apparent decline between 1848–54 and 1901 may have been due mainly to transfers to other categories (such as bronchitis, pneumonia, and influenza) as a result of improved certification. The other class of deaths which fell substantially was 'debility, atrophy and sudden death, cause unknown'.

The first two of these terms are quite unsatisfactory and the reduction of deaths was no doubt due largely to improvements in diagnosis and classification. Although violent deaths are shown separately in the Registrar-General's reports, those classified as sudden deaths may have included a considerable number caused by violence. About a quarter of these deaths were in the first year of life, so that some may have been due to infanticide. Others, no doubt ,were similar to those which would be described today as cot deaths, which means that the cause of death was unknown.

Against this background it seems reasonable to conclude that the Registrar-General's statistics provide no convincing evidence of a reduction of deaths from non-infective causes between 1848–54 and 1901, and the estimate of 8 per cent (Table 3.1) is probably due mainly to errors in certification and classification.

It would seem to follow that the fall of mortality before registration was associated almost entirely with infectious diseases. However, there are two non-infective causes of death (infanticide and starvation) which may have been important, although this cannot be confirmed from national statistics.

In a survey of the history of infanticide, Langer concluded that it was practised on a substantial scale in both ancient and modern times.[3] In the eighteenth and nineteenth centuries, 'the poor, hardly able to support the family they already had, evaded responsibility by disposing of further additions'. The same conclusion was reached by many contempory writers, among them Disraeli who believed that infanticide 'was hardly less prevalent in England than on the banks of the Ganges'. Langer also quoted Ryan who examined the medico-legal aspects of the problem of infanticide: 'We cannot ignore the fact that the crime of infanticide, as well as that of criminal abortion, is widespread and on the increase.' Although the frequency of infanticide cannot be estimated, there seems no reason to dissent from Langer's view that it was common until the last quarter of the nineteenth century, when it began to be reduced by stringent regulations, by growing public interest in maternal and child care, and finally and most effectively, by the spread of contraception.

It is also impossible to assess the frequency of death from starvation, as distinct from death from infectious diseases which resulted from poor nutrition. Although experience in developing countries today suggests

3. Langer W. L. 'Infanticide: a historical survey' *History of Childhood Quarterly*, **I** (1974), p. 353.

that the latter was much more common than the former, it seems probable that in the eighteenth and nineteenth centuries death did occur, perhaps not infrequently, as a direct result of food deficiency. In the first full year of registration of cause of death, 167 deaths were attributed to starvation. However, an analysis of 63 deaths by Farr showed that the classification was unsatisfactory (they included 12 persons who were said to have died from the effects of cold).

In spite of the lack of statistical evidence, I believe that death from infanticide was probably common, and death from starvation not uncommon, in the eighteenth and nineteenth centuries. If this is true, mortality from these causes may have declined before registration of cause of death in 1838, and certainly did so after that time. Although this trend cannot be confirmed from national statistics, it is quite possible that these were the only non-infective causes of death associated with a significant reduction of mortality before the twentieth century.

4

Infectious Diseases

I have concluded that the fall of mortality since the end of the seventeenth century was due predominantly to a reduction of deaths from infectious diseases. However, non-infective causes of death were associated with about a quarter of the decrease of deaths in this century. To understand the influences which have brought about the modern improvement in health it is therefore necessary to examine the reasons for the decline of the infections and of certain non-infective conditions. These are the subjects which will be discussed in this chapter and the one that follows.

This brings us to an important question in the history of the past three centuries. It will be suggested (Chapter 6) that the predominance of infectious diseases dates from the first agricultural revolution 10,000 years ago when men began to aggregate in populations of considerable size. Why then did the infections decline from about the time of the modern agricultural and industrial revolutions which led to the aggregation of still larger and more densely packed populations? The answer to this paradox must be sought in the character of micro-organisms, the conditions under which they spread and the response of the human host, inherited or acquired.

However, for an understanding of the infections it is unsatisfactory to consider separately an organism and its host. They are living things which interact and adapt to each other by natural selection. The virulence of an organism is not, therefore, a distinct character like its size or shape: it is an expression of an interaction between a particular organism and a particular host. For example, a measles virus, whose effects on children in a developed country are relatively benign, may have devastating effects when encountered by a population for the first time. When assessing the major influences on the infections it will therefore be necessary to distinguish between the following:

(*a*) Interaction between organism and host. When exposed to micro-organisms over a period of time, the hosts gain through natural selection an intrinsic resistance which is genetically determined. In addition to this intrinsic resistance immunity may also be acquired, by transmission from the mother or in response to a post-natal infection. These types of immunity, inherited and acquired, are not due to either medical intervention or, as a rule, to identifiable environmental influences.

(*b*) Immunization and therapy. Immunity may also result from successful immunization, and the outcome of an established infection may be modified by therapy.

(*c*) Modes of spread. These are very different for different micro-organisms, and the feasibility of control by preventing contact with an organism is determined largely by the way it is transmitted. In a developed country it is relatively easy to stop the spread of cholera by purification of water; it is more difficult to control salmonella infection by supervision of food-handling; and at present it is impossible to eliminate an airborne infection such as the common cold by preventing exposure to the virus.

(*d*) The nutrition of the host. The results of an encounter with a micro-organism are influenced not only by the inherited or acquired immunity of the host, but also by his general state of health determined particularly, it will be suggested, by nutrition.

This classification provides a basis for an analysis of reasons for the decline of infectious diseases. It is against the background of an understanding of the interaction between organism and host that we must consider the possibility that the decline was due substantially to a change in the character of the diseases, essentially independent of both medical intervention and identifiable environmental (including nutritional) improvements. It is in relation to immunization and therapy that we must assess the contribution of specific medical measures. A judgement on the significance of reduction of exposure to infection must rest on understanding of the modes of spread of micro-organisms. And an estimate of the importance of an increase in food supplies requires appraisal of the association between malnutrition and infection.

A CHANGE IN THE CHARACTER OF INFECTIOUS DISEASES

Was the decline of the infections during the past few centuries associated with a change in the character of the diseases, that is, with modification of the relation between the micro-organisms and their hosts? Such a change is not independent of the environment; indeed it is determined largely by an ecological relationship to the environment. It is, however, of a kind which must have occurred continuously during man's history.

It has been suggested that a change of this type was important, and even that it was the main reason for the decline of mortality and improvement in health. Greenwood, for example, emphasized the importance of the 'ever-varying state of the immunological constitution of the herd',[1] and in his presidential address to the American Association of Immunologists Magill wrote: 'It would seem to be a more logical conclusion that during recent years, quite regardless of our therapeutic efforts, a state of relative equilibrium has established itself between the microbes and the "ever-varying state of the immunological constitution of the herd"—a relative equilibrium which will continue, perhaps, just as long as it is not disturbed, unduly, by biological events.'[2] According to this interpretation, the trend of mortality from infectious diseases was essentially independent of both medical intervention and the vast economic and social developments of the past three centuries.

The grounds on which it was possible to reach so radical a conclusion are important. Magill based his views on the ineffectiveness and dangers of vaccination against rabies, the decline of tuberculosis long before effective treatment, the behaviour of diphtheria in the nineteenth century (it increased in prevalence and malignancy in the middle of the century and declined before the introduction of antitoxin), and the rapid reduction of pneumonia death-rates in New York State before the 'miracle' drugs were known, followed by an arrest of the decline from about the time when antibiotics were introduced. Moreover, these examples could be extended: the cholera vaccine required until recently by international regulations is almost useless; the reduction of mortality from diphtheria in the 1940s did not everywhere coincide with the introduction of immunization; and scarlet fever has had a variable history which appears to have been independent of medical and other influences.

Nevertheless, although specific measures had little effect on the trend of many infections, the question concerning the significance of changes

1. Greenwood, M. 'English death rates, past, present and future', *Journal of the Royal Statistical Society*, **99** (1936).
2. Magill, T. P., 'The immunologist and the evil spirits', *Journal of Immunology*, **74** (1955), 1.

in the character of the diseases is complex. It will therefore be desirable
to examine the implications of the suggestion that the decline of mortality was due substantially to a favourable change in the 'ever-varying
state of the immunological constitution of the herd'.

The immunological constitution of a generation is influenced largely
by the mortality experience of those which precede it. This was particularly true in the past, when the majority of live-born people died
from infectious diseases without reproducing. Under such conditions
there was rigorous natural selection in respect of immunity to infection.
The proposal that the decline of mortality resulted from a change in
the immunological constitution of the population therefore implies that
there was heavy mortality at an earlier period which led to the birth of
individuals who were genetically less susceptible. According to this
interpretation, the substantial and prolonged decline of infectious deaths
was due largely, not to improvements since the eighteenth century, but
to high mortality which must have preceded it.

AIRBORNE DISEASES

Although there is no airborne infection, indeed there is no infection,
of which it can be said that there has been no change in the relation
between organism and host since the eighteenth century, there are some
such as tuberculosis and, probably, measles in which it is unlikely to be
the main reason for the decrease of deaths. But the objection to this as
the main influence on all airborne infections is of a more general kind.
To believe that the reduction of deaths from these diseases was due
essentially to a change in their character, we should have to accept
either (a) that fortuitously, over the whole range of airborne diseases,
there was a change of the kind which appears to have occurred in
scarlet fever, independent of medical or other recognizable influences,
or (b) that certain deleterious influences led to high mortality in the
eighteenth century, which, through natural selection, resulted in the
survival of more resistant populations. In the light of the extent and
duration of the fall of mortality the first explanation is incredible. And
since there is no evidence that mortality from infectious diseases
increased greatly in the eighteenth century (on the contrary, there is
indirect evidence that it declined) the second explanation is equally
untenable.

WATER- AND FOOD-BORNE DISEASES

Although living conditions deteriorated in the first half of the nineteenth century, it is most unlikely that this led to the subsequent decline of mortality. In the first place, there is no evidence of a large increase of deaths from these diseases; and secondly, another and more plausible explanation is available, namely, improvements in hygiene (discussed below). This illustrates the advantages of separating water- and food-borne infections from those that are airborne. A change in the character of airborne diseases has to be considered in the light of the fact that exposure to the organisms cannot be prevented. But in the case of water- and food-borne diseases, separation from the source of infection was the critical step in their control. While, therefore, we cannot exclude the possibility that typhoid and dysentery at the end of the nineteenth century differed somewhat from the same diseases in the early industrial towns, it is unlikely that any difference was a major reason for the rapid decline of mortality from intestinal infections which followed improvements in water supply and sewage disposal.

VECTOR-BORNE DISEASES

As already noted, typhus is the vector-borne disease which may have contributed significantly to the fall of mortality in Britain, mainly in the eighteenth and early nineteenth centuries. As in the case of other epidemic infections, knowledge of the multiple factors which led to its disappearance and reappearance is still incomplete; but we cannot rule out the possibility that they included a change in the character of the disease, apparently unrelated to medical measures or identifiable environmental influences. However, even if the decrease of deaths from typhus could be accounted for largely in this way, its contribution to the decline of mortality would have been very small.

I conclude that the reduction of deaths from infectious diseases was not due substantially to a change in their character. This is not to suggest that it has not been modified, as in the case of scarlet fever and a few other less clear-cut examples. On the contrary, it is possible that genetically determined resistance to diseases such as tuberculosis and typhoid is lower today than it was in the eighteenth and nineteenth centuries. But if so, this has come about as a secondary consequence of reduced exposure, rather than through a primary change in the relation between the organisms and man. Moreover it is a change which, acting independently, would be expected to increase mortality rather than to reduce it.

IMMUNIZATION AND THERAPY

Until recently it was accepted, almost without question, that the modern improvement in health was due essentially to medical measures. However, this term is often used loosely in relation to both personal medical care and public health services; and since we are concerned here with the contribution of immunization and therapy (rather than our indebtedness to medical science in all its forms), it is important to distinguish between the two.

AIRBORNE DISEASES (see Table 3.3)

It is in respect of airborne diseases that assessment of the contribution of immunization and therapy is most important because (a) they were associated with the largest reduction of the death-rate (40.3 per cent) between 1848–54 and 1971 and (b) there is another obvious explanation for the decline of the water- and food-borne diseases which also contributed substantially.

Table 4.1 gives (in the second column) the proportion of the fall of the standardized death-rate associated with each disease or, in two cases, disease group. The table also shows the years when specific measures were introduced. The procedures referred to are as follows.

Tuberculosis: streptomycin, 1947. It is now well recognized that the methods of treatment in the first half of this century, for example pneumothorax and thorocoplasty, were of little value. The general use of BCG vaccination began later, in 1954.

Bronchitis, pneumonia, and influenza: sulphapyridine, 1938. Specific measures were ineffective before the introduction of the sulphonamides. The earliest (prontosil and sulphanilamide) were effective only against the streptococcus but trials of sulphapyridine suggested that it reduced mortality from lobar pneumonia. The scope of treatment was extended by the antibiotics which became available for civilian use about 1945.

Whooping cough: sulphonamides, 1938. Even today the effect of treatment by sulphonamides and antibiotics on the course of the disease is questionable. Immunization was used widely from 1952; the protective effect is variable, and has been estimated to lie between less than 20 per cent and more than 80 per cent.

TABLE 4.1. *Airborne diseases: fall of mortality since introduction of specific measures of prophylaxis or treatment: England and Wales*

Cause	Fall in standardized death-rate between 1848–54 and 1971 (a)	Fall as percentage of fall from all causes (b)	Year when specific measures became available	Fall by 1971 after introduction of specific measures (c)	Proportion of total fall after introduction of specific measures $\frac{c}{a}$	Fall after introduction of specific measures as percentage of total fall from all causes b/a
Tuberculosis (respiratory)	2,888	17.5	1947	409	0.14	2.5
Bronchitis, pneumonia, influenza	1,636	9.9	1938	531	0.32	3.2
Whooping cough	422	2.6	1938	43	0.10	0.3
Measles	342	2.1	1935	50	0.15	0.3
Scarlet fever } Diphtheria	1,016	6.2	{1935 1894	{15 292}	0.30	1.9
Smallpox	263	1.6	Before 1848	263	1.00	1.6
Infections of ear, pharynx, larynx	73	0.4	1935	, 65	0.89	0.4
	6,640	40.3	–	1,668	0.25	10.1

Measles: sulphonamides, 1935. Effective measures have only recently become available in the form of immunization and they had no significant effect on the trend of the death-rate. However, mortality from the disease is due largely to invasion by secondary organisms which have been treated by chemotherapy since 1935.

Scarlet fever: sulphonamides, 1935. There was no effective treatment before the introduction of prontosil.

Diphtheria: antitoxin, 1894. Antitoxin was used from the late nineteenth century and has been the accepted form of treatment since that time. Although questions have been raised about its effectiveness, it is generally believed to have lowered the case fatality rate, which fell from 8.2 per 100 notifications in 1916–25 to 5.4 in 1933–42, while notifications remained at an average level above 50,000 per year. The mortality rate increased at the beginning of the last war, but fell rapidly from about the time when national immunization was introduced.

Smallpox: vaccination, before 1848–54.

Infections of ear, pharynx, and larynx: sulphonamides, 1935. The main therapeutic influences have been chemotherapy and, in some ear infections, surgery. It is difficult to say exactly when surgical intervention became beneficial.

Table 4.1 shows the proportion of the reduction of mortality which occurred after the introduction of specific measures: about a quarter (0.25) of the fall from all airborne diseases and (as shown in the last column) about a tenth of that from all diseases (infective and non-infective).

The reduction of the death-rate attributable to immunization and therapy was of course much less than these figures suggest. Mortality from all the diseases was declining before, and in most cases long before, effective procedures became available. It is doubtful whether a reliable estimate can be made of the effect of medical intervention on the whole class of airborne diseases, but it is probably safe to conclude that they were not the main influence on the trend of mortality even from the time when immunization or treatment was introduced, except in the case of tuberculosis and diphtheria. Their contribution will be examined further in Chapter 8.

WATER- AND FOOD-BORNE DISEASES (see Table 3.4)

Cholera, diarrhoea, and dysentery. In the mid nineteenth century cholera was grouped with other diarrhoeal diseases in the Registrar-General's classification; however, the last epidemic in Britain was in 1865, and from that time the contribution of cholera was negligible. Mortality from the diarrhoeal diseases fell in the late nineteenth century; it increased between 1901 and 1911 but decreased rapidly from that time.

It is unlikely that treatment had any appreciable effect on the outcome of the diseases before the use of intravenous therapy in the 1930s, by which time 95 per cent of the improvement had occurred. For the main explanation of the fall of mortality we must look to the hygienic measures which reduced exposure.

Non-respiratory tuberculosis. Non-respiratory tuberculosis was an important cause of death in the nineteenth century. Although mortality fell quite rapidly after 1901, there was still a considerable number of deaths in England and Wales (197) in 1971.

Interpretation is complicated by the fact that non-respiratory tuberculosis is due to both human and bovine infections; the abdominal cases are predominantly bovine, whereas those involving bones and other organs are often caused by the human organism. The human types can be interpreted in the same terms as the pulmonary disease, but a different explanation must be sought for the bovine infection. It is unlikely that treatment contributed significantly to the fall of mortality, since the level was already low when streptomycin, the first effective measure, was introduced in 1947.

Typhoid and typhus. As noted in Chapter 3, mortality from typhus fell rapidly in the late nineteenth century and there have been few deaths in the twentieth. It can be said without hesitation that specific medical measures had no influence on this reduction.

The decline of enteric fevers was also rapid, and began before the turn of the century, somewhat earlier than the decrease of deaths from diarrhoea and dysentery. Effective treatment by chloramphenicol was not available until 1950, but by that time mortality from enteric fever was almost eliminated from England and Wales. Although immunization was used widely in the armed services during the war, its effectiveness is doubtful and it can have had little influence on the number of deaths.

In summary, the rapid decline of mortality from diseases spread by water and food since the late nineteenth century owed little to medical intervention. Immunization is relatively ineffective even today, and therapeutic measures of some value were not employed until about 1950, by which time the number of deaths had fallen to a low level.

OTHER DISEASES DUE TO MICRO-ORGANISMS (see Table 3.5)

Convulsions and teething. As mentioned previously, most of the deaths included under these unsatisfactory terms were due to infectious diseases of childhood, for example to whooping cough, measles, otitis media, meningitis, and gastro-enteritis. These infections are mainly airborne, and the general conclusions concerning the airborne diseases may be accepted for them. That is to say, it is unlikely that immunization and therapy had any significant effect on the frequency of death before the introduction of sulphonamides and antibiotics, and even after that time they were probably less important than other influences.

Syphilis. Although syphilis was associated with only 0.3 per cent of the reduction of mortality from the mid nineteenth century to 1971, it remained an important cause of sickness and death until about 1916, when salvarsan was made available without charge to medical practitioners. From this time the number of deaths fell, and was quite low in 1945 when penicillin largely replaced the arsenical preparations.

The decline of syphilis since its introduction to Europe in the fifteenth century was not due mainly to therapy, for after several centuries the disease had changed to a milder form. Nevertheless it seems right to attribute the fall of mortality since 1901 essentially to treatment. It should of course be recognized that effective treatment, as in the case of tuberculosis, not only benefits those affected by the disease, but also reduces the number of persons who spread the infection. It seems justified to regard this secondary effect as a further contribution of treatment.

Appendicitis, peritonitis. Mortality from these causes appeared to increase slightly during the nineteenth and early twentieth centuries, probably because of more accurate certification of cause of death, but declined after 1921. This improvement, which accounted for 0.4 per cent of the fall of the death-rate from all causes, can be attributed to treatment.

Puerperal fever. The death-rate from puerperal fever declined from the beginning of this century, but more rapidly after the introduction of the sulphonamides (1935) and, later, penicillin. It seems probable that the initial fall was due mainly to reduced exposure to infection during labour; but from 1935 the obstetric services were greatly strengthened by chemotherapy. Both influences can be credited to medical measures.

Other infections. The other conditions shown in Table 3.5 are a miscellaneous group, including some well recognized diseases which caused few deaths, either because they were uncommon in this period (as in the case of malaria, tetanus, poliomyelitis, and encephalitis) or because although common they were not often lethal (in the case of mumps, chicken pox, and rubella). They also include some relatively infrequent certified causes of death which are ill-defined, such as abscess, phlegmon, and pyaemia. In addition there is a very small number of deaths due to worm parasites which, strictly, do not belong among conditions due to micro-organisms.

These infections were associated with 3.5 per cent of the fall of mortality between the mid nineteenth century and 1971. In view of their varied aetiology it is not possible to assess accurately the major influences, but it is unlikely that therapy made much contribution before 1935. More than half of the reduction of deaths occurred before this time.

REDUCTION OF EXPOSURE TO INFECTION

Clearly, at least part of the decline of mortality from infectious diseases was due to reduced contact with micro-organisms. In developed countries an individual no longer meets the cholera vibrio, he is rarely exposed to the typhoid organism and he is infected by the tubercle bacillus much less often than in the past. But so far as can be judged there has been no considerable change in frequency of exposure to the streptococcus or the measles virus, and we must look elsewhere for an explanation of the decline of deaths from scarlet fever and measles.

The possibility of control of transmission of micro-organisms is determined largely by the ways they are spread. It is relatively easy (in developed countries) to prevent exposure to water-borne diseases; it is more difficult to control those spread by food, personal contact, and animal vectors; and it is usually impossible to prevent transmission of airborne infections.

AIRBORNE DISEASES

Since it is not possible to prevent transmission of airborne infections, it would seem to follow that reduction of exposure to them has played little part in the fall of mortality. However, this conclusion needs some qualification.

Although it is very difficult to prevent transmission of airborne diseases from one individual to another, less frequent exposure has nevertheless contributed to the decline of mortality from some infections. There are broadly two ways in which this has come about. The first is as a result of a reduction of prevalence; smallpox, syphilis, and tuberculosis are much less common than in the past, and exposure to them is correspondingly reduced. The second way is by improved living and working conditions, which prevent contact with infectious people in the community. However, these influences are not effective with all airborne diseases. In the case of a highly infectious condition such as measles, in communities in which it is endemic nearly all children became infected, in spite of improvements in living conditions and a large reduction in the number of serious cases.

In several of the airborne infections associated with the decline of mortality (Table 3.3) prevention of exposure has contributed little if anything to the decrease in the number of deaths. Although the death-rate from measles has fallen to a low level, infection rates remain high. There is no effective control of the organisms which cause bronchitis and pneumonia, and the influences which determine the disappearance and reappearance of the influenza virus are not well understood. The streptococcus, which is responsible for scarlet fever and for most of the infections of the ear, pharynx, and larynx, is ubiquitous, and the decline of these conditions owes little to reduced contact. However, in the case of the other diseases shown in Table 3.3 (tuberculosis, whooping cough, diphtheria, and smallpox) exposure to infection is undoubtedly less common than in the past. The change has come about, not as a primary influence, but as a secondary effect of other causes which reduced the prevalence of the diseases in the community. With the exception of smallpox and, possibly, tuberculosis, this influence was probably delayed until the twentieth century.

WATER- AND FOOD-BORNE DISEASES

It is in this class of diseases that a substantial reduction of mortality is likely to be achieved by prevention of exposure. The water- and food-borne diseases associated with the decline of the death-rate since the mid nineteenth century in England and Wales are shown in Table 3.4.

The death-rate from these diseases fell continuously from the second half of the nineteenth century. The exception is gastro-enteritis of infancy, whose decline was delayed until the twentieth century. There is no doubt that the fall of mortality from these diseases was due to reduced exposure brought about by improvements in hygiene.

For many years the decline of gastro-enteritis presented a problem (a central one in the interpretation of infant mortality) which arose from uncertainty about the infective nature of the disease. It is now clear that the provision of a safe milk supply was the main reason for the reduction of deaths from gastro-enteritis and contributed substantially to the fall of infant mortality from 1900.

The other water- and food-borne disease which contributed to the reduction of mortality was non-respiratory tuberculosis. The death-rate from the disease declined from 1848–54; considerably in the second half of the nineteenth century and even more rapidly after 1900. Although deaths due to human and bovine infections cannot be separated in national statistics, it seems probable that the human types were associated with the decline before 1900 and both types after 1900. In this case the fall of mortality in the nineteenth century can be discussed in the same terms as that of respiratory tuberculosis: it was not due to medical measures, or to a change in the character of the disease. The abdominal cases, however, were caused largely by infected milk, and their decline can be attributed to elimination of tuberculous cattle and to the more general measures taken to protect milk supplies after 1900.

OTHER DISEASES DUE TO MICRO-ORGANISMS

Most of the deaths shown under this heading were classified unsatisfactorily under convulsions and teething; several of them were undoubtedly due to airborne infections and their decline probably owed little to reduction of exposure. The infections (Table 3.5) which were affected were syphilis and puerperal fever, whose contributions to the fall of mortality were, however, very small. Moreover in the case of syphilis, less frequent exposure was a secondary result of treatment of the disease which decreased the number of infective persons, rather than a primary influence. In puerperal fever, exposure to infection was reduced by improved midwifery practice, following the teaching of Semmelweis.

Since reliable information about the diseases which declined in the eighteenth and early nineteenth centuries is not available, the possibility that exposure to infection was reduced at that time can only be assessed in general terms. Population growth and industrialization created optimum conditions for the spread of airborne infections, and if any reduction of exposure occurred it could have come about only as a secondary consequence of other influences which diminished the prevalence of the diseases in the community. It is in respect of the water- and food-borne diseases that the question of exposure is most important.

It is upon purification of water, efficient disposal of sewage and food hygiene that reduction of exposure to water- and food-borne diseases primarily depends. There are grounds for thinking that at least the first two of these influences deteriorated in the early nineteenth century when, under the pressure of population growth, the primitive sewage systems collapsed, and drinking water became more heavily polluted. It was not until the second half of the nineteenth century that these risks were largely controlled.

One can be less confident about the trend of food hygiene in the same period. What is clear is that there was little if any improvement in respect of milk, the most important component of the diet as a vehicle for transmission of disease. In an examination of the relation between milk supplies, infant mortality, and population growth, Beaver concluded that although the quantity of milk increased from the eighteenth century, it must have been heavily contaminated by pathogens.[3] It was not until the late nineteenth century that commercial pasteurization and bottling of milk were introduced, and not until the twentieth century that a safe supply became generally available.

Since most solid foods are protected, not by sterilization and sealing as in the case of milk, but by precautions in handling and distribution involving many people, it is not possible to say when the transition from an infected to a safe supply was achieved. However, it seems unlikely that food hygiene improved in the pre-registration period; indeed, it probably deteriorated, since the growth of towns made it necessary to transport large quantities of food from rural to urban areas, and thus resulted in increased handling and delayed consumption. A substantial advance in food hygiene was delayed until the present century, and rested largely on the work of microbiologists in the preceding fifty years.

3. Beaver, M. W., 'Population, infant mortality and milk', *Population Studies*, **27** (1973), 243.

Improvements in personal hygiene can also have had little influence on the trend of mortality, for as a defence against diseases such as typhoid and cholera when the water source is infected, the washing of hands is about as effective as the wringing of hands. The only reliable personal measures – boiling or chemical treatment of water – were unknown at that time. However, unwashed bodies and infrequently changed clothing and bedding provide ideal conditions for the body lice which carry typhus, and the low standards of cleanliness which prevailed before the nineteenth century no doubt contributed, perhaps substantially, to the prevalence of the disease. Standards began to improve in the late eighteenth century, first among the well-to-do, but later in all classes, and this change may have had some effect on the fall of mortality. However, the epidemiology of the disease is complex, and it is unlikely that any single influence accounted for its decline and eventual disappearance.

IMPROVEMENT IN NUTRITION

If the decline of mortality from infectious diseases was not due to a change in their character, and owed little to reduced exposure to micro-organisms before the second half of the nineteenth century or to immunization and therapy before the twentieth, the possibility that remains is that the response to infections was modified by an advance in man's health brought about by improved nutrition.

It should be said at once that there is no direct evidence that nutrition improved in the eighteenth and early nineteenth centuries. Evidence which could be regarded as convincing would be an increase in *per capita* food consumption or clinical observations showing an improvement in clinical state. These data do not exist, and few historical questions of such complexity would ever be resolved if they could be settled only by contemporary evidence of this kind. The case for the significance of nutrition is circumstantial. In this it is like the case for the origin of species by natural selection, which so far lacks confirmation by experimental production of a new species. It is nevertheless a convincing hypothesis because it has stood the test of critical examination in a variety of circumstances over an extended period. It is to a similar test that the suggestion concerning nutrition should be submitted.

The grounds for regarding better nutrition as the first and main reason for the reduction of infectious deaths are three-fold: this explanation is consistent with present-day experience of the relationship between

malnutrition and infection; it accounts for the fall of mortality and
growth of populations in many countries at about the same time; and
when extended to include improved hygiene and limitation of numbers, it attributes the decline of the infections to modification of the
conditions which led to their predominance.

MALNUTRITION AND INFECTIOUS DISEASE

It is well recognized that the health of an individual has a profound
bearing on his reaction to infectious disease. Measles is an example of
a condition in which infection rates are high in all social classes, but the
likelihood of serious illness and death depends largely on the health of
the child and is much increased among the poor. It is also clear that the
general state of health is determined by multiple influences, including
particularly previous illness and nutrition.

It is more difficult to go beyond these generalizations to a precise
estimate of the part played by nutrition in determining the outcome
of infectious disease. There are many conflicting reports in the literature,
and disorders of metabolism and deficiency diseases were accorded a
relatively minor role in the health of man and animals until recently.
However, Newberne and Williams have reviewed experimental evidence of nutritional influences on infections.[4] They suggested that the
effect of an infection depends to a considerable degree on the nutritional
condition of an animal at the time of exposure. A severe degree of
deficiency of almost any of the essential nutrients may have a marked
effect on the manner in which the host responds to an infectious agent.
The same infection may be mild or even inapparent in a well-nourished
animal, but virulent and sometimes fatal in one that is malnourished.
They refer to four ways in which nutrition influences infection:

(1) effects on the host which facilitate initial invasion of the infectious agent;
(2) through an effect on the agent once it is established in the tissues; (3) through
an effect on secondary infection; (4) by retarding convalescence after infection.

They concluded that

Grossly inadequate intakes of protein and other specific nutrients are today re-
sulting in extreme degrees of malnutrition and concomitant infectious disease.
It seems likely that the interactions between nutrition and infection are more

4. Newberne, P. M., and Williams, G., 'Nutritional influence on the course of
infections', in Dunlop, R. H., and Moon, H. W. (eds), *Resistance to Infectious
Disease* (Saskatoon Modern Press, 1970), p. 93.

important in animal and human populations than one would predict from the results of laboratory investigations. It must be remembered that the interaction between nutrition and infection is dynamic, being frequently characterized by synergism and less commonly by antagonism, and that control of malnutrition and infection are interdependent, so that the course of a disease is intimately related to the nutritional status of the host.

In man also it has proved difficult to obtain unequivocal results, for as food shortage and other features of poverty usually occur together, their respective contributions to mortality are hard to separate. For example, populations in which tuberculosis, or in a tropical country, schistosomiasis, are common are likely to be poor, underfed, and heavily exposed to infection; and it is not easy to determine the relative importance of malnutrition and frequent exposure. There is some evidence of a quasi-experimental kind in the increased incidence of infectious diseases in populations whose food intake was reduced substantially during the two world wars.

However, knowledge of the relation between malnutrition and infection has been extended considerably in recent years through experience of the World Health Organization in developing countries, where infectious diseases are still predominant. It leaves no doubt that although malnutrition does not have the same effect in every disease (for example, it is marked in diarrhoea, measles and tuberculosis, less so in whooping cough),[5] in general it is a major determinant of infection rates and of the outcome of infections. Moreover, infectious diseases have an unfavourable effect on nutritional state, and the interaction between disease and malnutrition leads to a vicious cycle which is characteristic of poverty and underdevelopment. These effects are not restricted to respiratory and intestinal infections for which there are no specific vaccines; mortality remains high from measles and whooping cough for which effective immunization is available, and indeed it is questionable whether infectious diseases can be controlled by vaccination in a malnourished population. The problems are particularly serious in infancy, before the child has developed its own natural defence mechanisms. The World Health Organization concluded that 'one half to three quarters of all statistically recorded deaths of infants and young children are attributed to a combination of malnutrition and infection'.[6] The

5. Morley, D., *Paediatric Priorities in the Developing World* (London, 1973), pp. 184, 217, 238, 259.
6. World Health Organization, *Better Food for a Healthier World*, Features, FS/19 (1973).

deficiency is due mainly to lack of calories and proteins, although mineral and vitamin deficiencies are frequently associated.

It should be emphasized that the malnutrition which is the common background of infectious diseases in developing countries is not necessarily, and is not usually of the overt types such as rickets, beri-beri, pellagra, and the protein-calorie deficiency syndromes, kwashiorkor and marasmus; it is more often manifested as chronic malnutrition without specific features. This no doubt explains why it was unrecognized in previous centuries. Two-thirds of the populations of some countries are estimated to suffer from this less obvious kind of deficiency, in which infection is frequently the final influence which results in death. The interpretation of this experience was discussed in a recent report from the World Health Organization.

A debilitated organism is far less resistant to attacks by invading micro-organisms. Ordinary measles or diarrhoea—harmless and short-lived diseases among well-fed children—are usually serious and often fatal to the chronically malnourished. Before vaccines existed, practically every child in all countries caught measles, but 300 times more deaths occurred in the poorer countries than in the richer ones. The reason was not that the virus was more virulent, nor that there were fewer medical services; but that in poorly nourished communities the microbes attack a host which, because of chronic malnutrition, is less able to resist. The same happens with diarrhoea, respiratory infections, tuberculosis and many other common infections to which malnourished populations pay a heavy and unnecessary toll.[7]

The same report gave the results of a recent investigation of mortality in infancy in Latin America, which concluded that 'when malnutrition was not given as the major cause of death in official statistics, it was an associated cause in 50–80 per cent of cases. Malnutrition was also a concomitant factor in 60 per cent of the deaths attributable to measles'. The author concluded that malnutrition was the most serious health problem among the populations studied.

These and other investigations show the enormous importance of nutrition in determining the outcome of infection, and the tragic synergistic relation which exists between malnutrition and infectious disease. The World Health Organization report suggested that 'we have given too much attention to the enemy and have to some extent overlooked our own defences'. That is to say we have concentrated on specific measures such as vaccination and environmental improvement without

7. Behar, M., 'A deadly combination', *World Health* (February–March, 1974), p. 29.

sufficient regard for the predominant part played by nutritional state.
'For the time being,' it concluded, 'an adequate diet is the most effective
"vaccine" against most of the diarrhoeal, respiratory and other common
infections.'

CONCOMITANT GROWTH OF POPULATIONS

The rapid growth of populations in a large number of countries which
differed in economic and other conditions (the United States, England
and Ireland are remarkable examples) has led some historians to conclude that no single explanation is likely to be adequate. The opposite
conclusion seems more plausible: the widespread expansion of numbers
in many countries at about the same time in spite of variation in circumstances suggests the possible operation of a common major change.

The increase in food supplies which resulted from advances in agriculture and transport in the eighteenth and nineteenth centuries was
such a change. Although early estimates of food production were unreliable, there is no doubt that it increased. In eighteenth-century
Britain, for example, grain and meat production seems to have at least
kept pace with the growth of population, and in some years there was
a small surplus for export. During the last years of the century there
was a succession of poor harvests, which led to widespread food short-
ages and forced the government to prohibit the export of grain and to
lift the existing ban on animal imports from Ireland. These difficulties
were temporary, and during the first half of the nineteenth century both
the amount of land devoted to cereal production and the yield per acre
continued to increase. In 1840, the quantity of imported wheat relative
to total consumption was no more than it had been in 1811 (about 5 per
cent). After 1885, however, imports of wheat and other foods rose
substantially, and by 1870 about a fifth of the nation's food came from
abroad.

The most impressive evidence of the improvement in food supplies
is, therefore, the fact that the expanded populations were fed essentially
on home-grown food. The population of England and Wales increased
from 5.5 million in 1702 to 8.9 in 1801 and 17.9 in 1851. Since exports
and imports of food during this period were relatively small, it is clear
that food production at least trebled to sustain an increase of 12.4
million in a century and a half.

The effect of the additional food on population growth in a country would of course be determined by many variables, particularly the initial levels of fertility and mortality, the subsequent behaviour of the birth-rate and the amount of migration. Hence the variation between countries in the extent and timing of the increase in numbers does not exclude the possibility that the reduction of mortality was first and for some time due to improvement in nutrition.

CONTROL OF CAUSES OF INFECTIONS

Perhaps the most important requirement in a credible explanation for the decline of infectious diseases is that it should take account of the reasons for their predominance; we cannot be satisfied with an interpretation which suggests that the conditions which made them the common causes of sickness and death for ten thousand years remained essentially unchanged. This would be the case if immunization and therapy were the major influences during the past three centuries; or if mortality had fallen largely because of a reduction of virulence of micro-organisms. Moreover, if these were the reasons for the decline of the infections, we could be anything but confident about their future control. For in the light of experience of drug resistance we cannot foresee the long-term consequences of immunization and therapy; and if infectious deaths decreased because of a fortuitous change in virulence, they could quite readily increase again for the same reason.

The interpretation outlined in Chapter 6 attributes the predominance of infectious diseases since the first agricultural revolution to the expansion and aggregation of populations, poor hygiene and insufficient food; and their decline to modification or removal of these influences, spread over more than two centuries. During industrialization, however, the aggregation of populations increased; and in the early stages the hygiene, to put it cautiously, did not improve. It is therefore impressive that a large increase in food supplies coincided with population growth in many countries which differed widely in economic and other conditions. Of course, it is arguable that the expanded populations consumed all the additional food, so that there was no *per capita* increase. But in view of the other circumstantial evidence, as well as the lack of substance in alternative explanations, it seems more likely that at a time when birth-rates and death-rates were high, the population expanded because better nutrition resulted in increased resistance to infectious diseases, particularly in infants and children.

Before ending this discussion of nutrition I should consider briefly a possible objection, that there was a substantial increase in life-expectation of the aristocracy during the eighteenth and nineteenth centuries, although it is unlikely that well-to-do people offered much scope for improvement in nutrition. If we can accept that their expectation of life did increase, and one hesitates to rely on statistical data for the period before births and deaths were recorded nationally, two possible explanations can be considered.

One is that in the eighteenth and nineteenth centuries, when the prevalence of infectious desease was declining in the general population, all sections benefited from the secondary effects of reduced exposure. This possibility is well illustrated by experience of tuberculosis in the past century. The disease occurred in wealthy people, although less often and less seriously than among the poor. The difference between the social classes was determined partly by different levels of exposure, but also by the better nutrition of the well-to-do which reduced both the frequency and the severity of the illness. Nevertheless, mortality from tuberculosis undoubtedly declined in the middle and upper classes, as in the population as a whole, long before the introduction of effective treatment in 1947. It did so, presumably, because the disease had become less prevalent in the community as a result of a general advance in nutrition. Thus well-to-do people benefited from a secondary effect of improved nutrition.

A further possibility is that there was a primary reduction of exposure to infection, particularly in early childhood. For the newborn the cleanliness of food is critical, and while the children of the aristocracy no doubt had sufficient food, standards of hygiene probably left a good deal to be desired. The transfer of the care of infants to wet-nurses meant that standards of care were often little better than those of the population at large. Although the condition of water supplies did not improve until the second half of the nineteenth century, and the cleanliness of food not until the beginning of the twentieth, it is possible that the standards of personal hygiene of well-to-do people improved from the late eighteenth century; certainly they used amenities such as water-closets long before they became available to the general public. But these suggestions are inevitably tentative, and it is questionable whether it will ever be possible to be confident about social class differences in health experience before they can be verified in national statistics.

5

Non-Infective Conditions

The evidence for England and Wales suggests that with the possible exceptions of infanticide and starvation, about which information is lacking, non-infective causes of death were not associated with the decline of mortality before 1900. In the twentieth century, however, the reduction of deaths from non-infective conditions was considerable; moreover it has been concealed to some extent by the increase in mortality from lung cancer and myocardial infarction, brought about by smoking and other influences. In this brief examination of reasons for the decline of non-infective deaths the effect of these increases will be ignored (it would be very difficult to take account of them) and the causes of death associated with the decline will be referred to in order according to their contribution to the reduction of mortality.

DEATHS IN THE TWENTIETH CENTURY

Much of the largest fall (1,057 deaths per million between 1901 and 1971) was associated with the heterogeneous class, 'prematurity, immaturity and other diseases of infancy'. These deaths were almost restricted to the first year of life, and their contribution to the decline of infant mortality was of the same order of magnitude as that of deaths due to an infection: gastro-enteritis. In 1901 more than 90 per cent of them were certified under two headings, 'premature birth' and 'atrophy, debility'. The latter no longer appears in the Registrar-General's classification, so that the large decrease in the number of deaths is explained by transfers to other causes, many of which have of course declined. Premature birth had no consistent meaning in 1901; it was later identified with low birth-weight until the internationally agreed basis was changed, to take account of the duration of gestation. With due regard for these inconsistencies, there has undoubtedly been a large reduction in deaths of this type in the first year of life. This contribution to the fall of the non-infective death-rate was probably due in part to a rising standard of living, particularly improvement in maternal nutrition which lowered the incidence of premature birth, and in part to improved obstetric care (before and during labour) and better management of the premature infant.

Nothing more need be said about deaths attributed to 'old age' in 1901, whose rapid decline was evidently due to transfers to more satisfactory diagnoses. Next in magnitude (according to their contribution to the fall of the death-rate in the twentieth century) were 'other diseases', which comprised a considerable number of causes of death, many of which would today be unacceptable. The largest reductions were associated with alcoholism, rickets, and non-infective diseases of the respiratory system other than emphysema and asthma, and are probably explained in part by less frequent drinking, improved nutrition, and, particularly in the case of the respiratory diseases, better certification. There were also some causes of death (for example, eczema) whose decline was no doubt largely due to treatment.

'Other diseases of digestive system' exclude cancers, but include some causes of death whose decrease was due to better certification (for example, gastric catarrh). The largest reductions appear to have been associated with conditions now treated by surgery (gall bladder disease, hernia, and intestinal obstruction) and with cirrhosis whose decline is attributable to less frequent drinking.

The next two classes, rheumatic heart disease* and nephritis, are essentially infective and are misplaced in this discussion. They have been included only because Table 3.6 examined the trend of mortality in the nineteenth as well as the twentieth century, and for 1848–54 these infections cannot be separated from non-infective causes of death. To this extent the estimate of the contribution of non-infective conditions to the fall of the death-rate is overstated.

There seems little doubt that the decline of mortality from violence in the twentieth century, when the frequency of accidents has risen steadily, was due predominantly to surgery.

The deaths under 'other diseases of nervous system' include brain tumour, diseases of the cord and neuritis, where the diagnoses must be in doubt. The improvement was mainly in respect of epilepsy, and may be attributed to treatment. The reasons for the reduction of the death-rate from cerebrovascular disease are not clear, and the contributions of

---

* In Table 3.6, rheumatic heart disease is included under cardiovascular disease.

the two remaining classes (other diseases of urinary system and pregnancy and childbirth, excluding sepsis) were small.

From this brief analysis it is evident that interpretation of the trend
of non-infective causes of death can be attempted only in very general
terms; the influences are more varied and less specific than in the case
of the infections. Therapeutic measures made a substantial contribution
in respect of some causes of death; for example there is little doubt
about the value of surgery in cases of violence and in several digestive
disorders. It is not possible to be equally confident about the effects of
treatment on some other conditions listed in Table 3.6. The heterogeneous class of deaths ascribed to prematurity, immaturity, other
diseases of infancy made the largest contribution to the total decline of
mortality. These deaths were almost restricted to the first year of life,
and their reduction, together with that of deaths due to gastro-enteritus,
was the main reason for the rapid fall of infant mortality from the
beginning of the century. While this trend no doubt owed something
to improvements in obstetric services, before and during labour, it was
probably due mainly to advances in maternal nutrition and better infant
feeding and care. Some of the decline shown in Table 3.6 was associated
with changes in classification of causes of death, and in two cases at
least (rheumatic fever and nephritis) was due to inclusion of what were
essentially infective conditions.

DEATHS BEFORE THE TWENTIETH CENTURY

INFANTICIDE

I referred above to Langer's review of the history of infanticide, which
suggested that it was practised on a substantial scale, at least until the
second half of the nineteenth century, and probably in some developing
countries until the present day.[1] Although this conclusion cannot be
confirmed by national statistics, for obvious reasons, it is nevertheless
consistent with extensive historical evidence assembled by Langer and
others. That infanticide remained common at least until the late nineteenth century is suggested by the fact that R. L. Stevenson and his
family were surprised to find that there were few children in the
populations they encountered on the islands in the Pacific.

But although infanticide was probably common in the eighteenth

1. Langer, W. L., op. cit., p. 353.

and previous centuries, it is not possible to say exactly when the practice declined. It seems likely that it became less frequent as the growth of foundling hospitals made it possible for a mother to get rid of an unwanted child rather than destroy it. This development is well illustrated by the experience of a foundling hospital in St Petersburg:

By the mid 1830s it had 25,000 children on its rolls and was admitting 5000 newcomers annually. Since no questions were asked and the place was attractive, almost half of the new-born babies were deposited there by their parents. A dozen doctors and 600 wet-nurses were in attendance to care for the children during the first six weeks, after which they were sent to peasant nurses in the country. At the age of six (if they survived to that age) they were returned to St Petersburg for systematic education. The programme was excellent, but its aims were impossible to achieve. Despite all excellent management and professional efforts, thirty to forty per cent of the children died during the first six weeks and hardly a third reached the age of six.[2]

In England, Parliament (1756) made provision for asylums for exposed or deserted young children to be opened in all counties, ridings, and divisions of the kingdom; and in France, Napoleon in 1811 decreed that there should be hospitals in every department. However, the demand was far beyond the resources of the foundling institutions, and it was not until the last quarter of the nineteenth century that the practice of infanticide became uncommon and not until the twentieth that (in western Europe) it virtually disappeared. Its decline occurred over approximately the same period as the fall of the birth-rate, and while many other developments may have contributed (for example improved living conditions and maternal and child welfare services) the main influence was undoubtedly the growth of contraceptive practices which reduced the number of unwanted births.

STARVATION

This is another non-infective cause of death which may have declined significantly in the pre-registration period and later. Again, statistical evidence is deficient. Moreover, as noted in the preceding chapter, unless food supplies are very inadequate, there are many more cases of chronic malnutrition associated with infectious diseases but without definitive signs, than there are cases (such as rickets or kwashiorkor) with specific evidence of deficiency or frank starvation. But if it is

2. Langer, W. L., op. cit., p. 358.

accepted that the nutrition of the population was poor at the beginning of the eighteenth century and has improved continuously since that time, it seems likely that some people must have been at or near starvation level and that their numbers decreased. This conclusion is not difficult to accept for the eighteenth and nineteenth centuries, when it is recognized that in the wealthiest countries there are people who are underfed even in the present day.

I conclude that the decline of mortality from non-infective causes of death (infanticide and starvation in the eighteenth and nineteenth centuries and a large number of conditions in the twentieth) was due partly to medical measures, but also to contraception and improvement in nutrition. Indeed, since the reduction of deaths from infanticide probably made the largest contribution to the decline, the change in reproductive behaviour which resulted in avoidance of unwanted pregnancies may have been the most important influence on the decrease of deaths from non-infective conditions.

6

Health in the Past

The preceding chapters were concerned with the modern improvement in health, as indicated by the reduction of deaths from infective and non-infective causes during the past three centuries. We must now consider, in the light of the conclusions drawn in these chapters, the nature of the disease problems and of the influences – nutritional, environmental, behavioural and therapeutic – that have been at work at different times in man's history to the present day.

There are various ways in which history might be divided for this purpose, for example, in relation to economic conditions (poverty and affluence), or by the nature of the common diseases (infectious and non-communicable). But perhaps the most instructive division is according to way of life: four periods or phases can be identified – nomadic, agricultural, transitional and industrial – each of which is characterized by certain predominant disease problems. Because the industrial period is typical of the future rather than the past, it will be discussed separately in Chapter 7.

THE NOMADIC PERIOD

During most of his time on earth, indeed for all but about the last ten-thousandth, man has lived as a nomad, dependent for his food on hunting, fishing and gathering fruit. Under such conditions the earth supports no more than a few people per square mile, and it has been estimated that when cultivation and domestication of plants and animals began about 10,000 years ago, the total population was below, and probably well below, 10 million. It is generally believed that life was short, and it would seem to follow that the slow rate of population growth was due to high mortality.

However, this conclusion has been questioned. It has been suggested that primitive man may have been able to restrict fertility, by such means as abstinence, contraception, abortion and prolonged lactation, so that numbers born were limited to levels that could be supported by the resources of the environment. It is generally accepted that mortality was relatively high, but this is attributed to hunting accidents and tribal wars rather than to lack of essentials such as food. Life, though short, was thought to be comparatively healthy.

The belief that the fertility of early man was effectively restrained is influenced largely by the suggestion that a similar mechanism operates widely among animals in their natural habitats.[1] This conclusion has been criticized on several grounds,[2] of which the most compelling is that it is based on the concept of 'group selection', the idea that by restricting fertility animal populations maintain themselves 'at about the level at which food resources are utilized to the fullest extent possible without depletion'.[1] Since this implies that the majority of those born alive survive and reproduce, it is clearly in conflict with the Darwinian concept of natural selection. For group selection, if widely practised, would reduce the ability of living things to adapt to a changing environment through high fertility followed by high and selective mortality.

The main causes of death among animals in their natural habitats are food shortage, disease and predation. According to Lack, 'the numbers of most birds, carnivorous mammals, certain rodents, large fish where not fished and a few insects are limited by food'.[3] Numbers of some other animals, including gallinaceous birds, for most of the time are limited by predators, including insect parasites. But since predation results from the need for food, it is food supplies which directly through starvation or indirectly through predation determine the level of mortality and limit population size.

In view of the prominence of infectious disease in man in recent centuries, it is important to note that this is not a common cause of death in birds and other wild animals. Population sizes and densities of most animals are probably too low to maintain micro-organisms in the absence of an intermediate host. However, there are exceptions, particularly among arthropods, and it is significant that insects – the most numerous of the world's animal species – appear to have a central place in the history of viruses.

The levels of fertility and mortality and the causes of death of early man are of course unknown, and it is questionable whether the observations

1. Wynne-Edwards, V. C., op. cit., p. 132.
2. Lack, D., op. cit., p. 300.
3. Lack, D., op. cit., p. 287.

that have been made on the few peoples who have retained a primitive way of life to the present day have much bearing on the main issues. However, it is possible to judge the feasibility of limiting births in the absence of modern knowledge and techniques. A minimum weight for height is essential for the onset and maintenance of regular menstruation, so it is quite likely that fertility was often relatively low, as in some developing countries today, because of the prevalence of malnutrition. It is unlikely that early man was able to control numbers by intentionally restricting fertility. In developing countries there is no evidence of effective control by the practice of continence or, until recently, contraception; both experimental and epidemiological findings indicate that prolonged lactation is not a reliable means of avoiding pregnancy; and it is only in recent years in medical hands that abortion has become a safe and effective instrument. The method of undoubted effectiveness frequently discussed in this context is infanticide, but this is a post-natal rather than a prenatal influence.

If restraints on the fertility of early man were ineffective, except for the involuntary one imposed by insufficient food, it follows that the growth of the world's population was restricted by high mortality. This conclusion is consistent with the experience of developing countries today and of advanced countries in the recent past.

The common causes of death probably fell broadly into two classes, the first comprising those for which man was responsible (all forms of homicide, including infanticide and tribal war) and those for which he was not directly responsible (food deficiency, disease and injuries arising from hunting and gathering). On the evidence available, or likely to become available, it is impossible to assess the relative contributions of these influences, which no doubt varied from one population to another and from time to time. What can be said is that all of them are related to the environment, and particularly to food supplies. For if homicide in its various forms was common, it was presumably determined ultimately by limitations of resources. And if starvation or disease associated with food deficiency were important, they resulted even more directly from lack of food.

Viewed in this way, the causes of death were analogous to those outlined by Lack in his interpretation of the experience of other animals. At times mortality was probably due mainly to shortage of food and associated disease; at other times food limits may not have been reached because of a high death-rate from causes such as infanticide and tribal war. This is consistent with the conclusion that the main restraint on population growth was a high level of mortality determined directly or indirectly by lack of food.

As noted above, infectious disease is not a common cause of death of animals in their natural habitats, and the same is probably true of early man. He may have suffered from infections of which precursors are found in other primates, and from some contracted from animal vectors; but living in small groups he is unlikely to have experienced many of the diseases which were later prominent, particularly those that are airborne (such as measles, mumps, smallpox, tuberculosis, influenza, diphtheria and the common cold). Among modern amenities for which our ancestors had little need was the pocket handkerchief.

THE AGRICULTURAL PERIOD

There have been two major changes from the conditions of life of early man and both had profound effects on health and population growth. The first occurred with the transition from a nomadic to a settled way of life; the second was associated with the agricultural and industrial developments of the last three centuries. Although we are concerned here mainly with the modern period, it is essential as a background to understand the effects of the earlier changes.

The first agricultural revolution brought an increase in food supplies which led to a decline of mortality and expansion of numbers. Why then, after an initial spurt, did the world's population rise so slowly that it was not until 1830 that it reached 1,000 million? The answer to this question must be sought in man's experience of infectious disease at different periods of his history.

To interpret experience of the infections it is necessary to recognize that micro-organisms and man have evolved in balance, and the relationship is constantly changing through the operation of natural selection in parasite and host. Hence changes in the character of the infections proceed continuously, and although related to the environment are largely independent of recognizable influences. Moreover, the stability of the relationship is different for different organisms; for example, it is very variable in the case of the streptococcus, but less so in that of the tubercle bacillus or measles virus.

While man lived as a nomad, infection was not the predominant cause of sickness and death. It became so 10,000 years ago as a result of the expansion and aggregation of populations which created the condition required for the propagation and transmission of micro-organisms.

However, as population growth was uncontrolled, numbers increased to the point where food resources again became marginal, so that the relation between man and micro-organisms causing disease evolved over a period when man was, in general, poorly nourished. The relationship was unstable and finely balanced according to the physiological state of host and parasite; an improvement in nutrition would tip the balance in favour of the former, and a deterioration in favour of the latter. In these circumstances an increase in food supplies became a necessary condition for a substantial reduction of mortality from infectious diseases, and limitation of numbers would have to follow if the reduction was to be made permanent. These were critical advances made in the western world in the eighteenth and nineteenth centuries.

THE TRANSITIONAL PERIOD

The period from about the beginning of the eighteenth century to the present day was one of change from an agricultural to an industrial way of life. In the most advanced countries the transition has been largely achieved; but in some developing areas it has scarcely begun, and on a world view it will not be completed until some time in the next century. What is particularly significant is that in developed countries there have also been profound changes in economic conditions, from poverty to affluence, and in the character of the common disease problems, from infections to non-communicable diseases. Hence in the transitional period, both within countries and between countries, there is a mix of health problems, since those that were predominant in the past exist side by side with those that will be predominant in the future.

The influences that are bringing about this change were examined in Chapters 3–5, and it will be necessary only to summarize the conclusions.

The first and most important reason for the decline of infectious diseases was an improvement in nutrition. It resulted from advances in agriculture which spread throughout the western world from about the end of the seventeenth century. Although incidental to our theme, it is of great interest that the advance was due initially to the introduction of new crops such as the potato and maize, and to more effective application of traditional methods – increased land use, manuring, winter feeding, rotation of crops, etc. – rather than to mechanical or chemical methods associated with industrialization. In the beginning, therefore, the Industrial Revolution did not create its own labour force, since the decline of mortality and growth of population preceded it and were, for some time after it began, essentially independent of it. However, from the second half of the nineteenth century agricultural productivity was greatly increased by the introduction of mechanization and the use of chemical fertilizers and, later, pesticides.

Second only to nutritional influences, in time and probably in importance, were the improvements in hygiene introduced progressively from the second half of the nineteenth century. They were the predominant reasons for the decline of water- and food-borne diseases, associated with about a fifth of the reduction of mortality from all causes between the mid nineteenth century and the present day (Table 3.2). The questions related to this influence which need a little further attention are its timing and character.

For the period since cause of death was registered we are on fairly secure ground in dating the advance from about 1870 in England and Wales; it was somewhat later in most other countries. The reduction of deaths from intestinal infections began at this time, and coincided with improvements initiated by sanitary reformers. There are no data that enable us to judge the trend of intestinal infections before registration of cause of death; but with an expanding population hygiene is unlikely to have advanced in the eighteenth century, and after the movement to towns, with uncontrolled living and working conditions, it must have deteriorated. Hence we can be fairly confident that reduction of exposure to infection, through better hygiene, was delayed until the 1870s, although there may well have been some improvement as a secondary consequence of the declining prevalence of disease at an earlier period.

There is also little doubt about the character of the hygienic measures. In the nineteenth century there were no large improvements in working and living conditions, and the main advances were in purification of water and sewage disposal. From about 1900 these measures were greatly extended by food hygiene, affecting most critically the quality of milk. Before that time it was not possible to protect milk from micro-organisms, and the rapid fall of deaths from gastro-enteritis, which contributed substantially to the decline of infant mortality, was due to the introduction of sterilization, bottling, and safe transport of milk. Environmental measures have of course been extended in the present century, by improvements in working and living conditions, taking the latter to include advances (such as control of atmospheric pollution) in the community at large as well as in domestic circumstances.

The conclusions concerning the influence of immunization and therapy on the infections may be summarized as follows. Except in the case of vaccination against smallpox (associated with 1.6 per cent of the reduction of the death-rate in England and Wales from 1848–54 to 1971), it is unlikely that personal medical care had a significant effect on mortality from infectious diseases before the twentieth century. Between 1900 and 1935 there was a contribution in some diseases: antitoxin in treatment of diphtheria; surgery in appendicitis, peritonitis, and ear infections; salvarsan in syphilis; intravenous therapy in diarrhoeal diseases; passive immunization against tetanus; and improved obstetric care in prevention of puerperal fever. But even if these measures were responsible for the whole decline of mortality from these conditions after 1900, which clearly they were not, they would account for only a small part of the decrease of deaths which occurred before 1935. From that time the first powerful chemotherapeutic agents, sulphonamides and, later, antibiotics, came into use, and they were supplemented by improved vaccines. However, they were certainly not the only reasons for the continued fall of mortality. I conclude that immunization and treatment contributed little to the reduction of deaths from infectious diseases before 1935, and over the whole period since cause of death was first registered they were much less important than other influences.

In the light of these conclusions concerning the twentieth century, it is most unlikely that personal medical care had a significant effect on the trend of mortality in the eighteenth and early nineteenth centuries.

The other reason for the modern transformation of health was the change in reproductive behaviour which led to the decline of the birth-rate. The significance of this change can hardly be exaggerated. In England and Wales, for example, if the birth-rate had continued at its earlier level, the population today would be about 140 rather than 50 million. The effects on health and welfare can be imagined. While, therefore, the initial progress was due to other influences, the change in reproductive practices which restricted numbers was the essential complement without which the advances, like those associated with the first agricultural revolution, would soon have been reversed.

Moreover, the restraint on reproduction probably had a direct effect on mortality. If infanticide had the significance which has been suggested, the virtual elimination of this important cause of death was due mainly to avoidance of unwanted pregnancies. Indeed, as noted previously, it is quite possible that this behavioural change made the largest contribution to the decline of non-infective causes of death.

It would be unwise to attempt to express numerically the contribution that different influences have made to the fall of mortality. There are too many unknowns. We do not know the causes of death in the eighteenth and early nineteenth centuries, so conclusions for that time can only be informed guesses. Since registration of cause of death, the Registrar-General's classification has included some ill-defined and heterogeneous categories (such as 'prematurity, immaturity, other diseases of infancy' and 'old age') whose composition is far from clear. And it is not possible to estimate with any precision the contribution which therapeutic and other advances have made to the decline of the multiple non-infective causes of death which together were associated with about a quarter of the reduction of mortality in this century.

With due regard for these and other grounds for reservation, I believe it is possible to draw a few general conclusions concerning the main influences on health during the past three centuries.

1. Improvement in nutrition was the earliest, and, over the whole period since about 1700, the most important influence.

2. Hygienic measures were responsible for at least a fifth of the reduction of the death-rate between the mid nineteenth century and today. This is the proportion of the decline which was associated with water- and food-borne diseases.

3. With the exception of vaccination against smallpox, whose contribution was small, the influence of immunization and therapy on the death-rate was delayed until the twentieth century, and had little effect on national mortality trends before the introduction of sulphonamides in 1935. Since that time it has not been the only, or, probably, the most important influence.

4. The change in reproductive practice which led to the decline of the birth-rate was very significant, since it ensured that the improvement in health brought about by other means was not reversed by rising numbers.

If we group together the advances in nutrition and hygiene as environmental measures, the influences responsible for the decline of mortality and increased expectation of life were environmental, behavioural and therapeutic. They became effective from the eighteenth, nineteenth and twentieth centuries respectively, and their order in time was also that of their effectiveness.

7

Health in the Future

The appraisal of influences on health in the past three centuries suggested that we owe the improvement, not to what happens when we are ill, but to the fact that we do not so often become ill; and we remain well, not because of specific measures such as vaccination and immunization, but because we enjoy a higher standard of nutrition and live in a healthier environment. In at least one important respect, reproduction, we also behave more responsibly.

However, it is unlikely that these influences will have the same relative importance in the future. In industrialized countries the decline of the infections has been followed by a change in the character of health problems; and even in developing countries it is possible that the influences have been modified by advances in medicine and in science and technology in general. It is therefore worth examining the nature of the residual problems which are becoming predominant as the infections decline.

RESIDUAL HEALTH PROBLEMS

From the discussion of the determinants of health (Chapter 2) it is evident that there are only two ways in which disease occurs. It results either from errors in genetic programming at fertilization, or from the fact that the embryo, foetus or live-born individual, correctly programmed, is exposed to an environment for which the genes are not adapted. Haemophilia and Turner's syndrome are examples of the first mechanism; most congenital malformations and the common types of physical and mental illness appear to be examples of the second.

If a proposition in this form (everything is A or is not A) seems self-evident, its implications for our understanding of disease origins are not. In the first place, the environment (using the term in reference to all non-hereditary influences) for which the genes are adapted is not that of the present day, but the one in which our ancestors evolved during the hundreds of thousands of years of the nomadic period. The requirements for health of the digestive, cardiovascular and reproductive systems are therefore likely to be that the demands on them should not differ greatly from those made during man's evolution. When confronted with the uncertainties of evidence relating diet, exercise and reproductive experience to diseases of these systems, it is instructive to ask ourselves in what ways present-day practices have departed from those of early man. For example, one can see why nutritionists tell us that we may eat what we like so long as we don't like much – particularly saturated fats, sugar in its various forms, some animal proteins, coffee, alcohol, refined foods and unrefined foods which have been made palatable by additives. These restrictions are severe, but understandable, when we realize that their aim is to bring us nearer to the dietary regime of our ancestors who were hungry most of the time.

There is a further consideration, namely, that vast changes from the conditions under which man evolved were associated with the transitions from nomadic to agricultural to industrial ways of life. At the risk of some oversimplification, it might be said that both the nomadic and the agricultural periods were characterized by the multiple effects of poverty whose influence in health was aggravated by lack of knowledge; but the later period differed from the earlier in the predominance of infectious diseases. Industrialization, with the advances in agriculture and increased knowledge of disease origins and mechanisms, brought relief from many of the problems associated with poverty; but by providing an excess of resources over needs, it opened the way to the ill-effects of affluence.

However, except in relation to some infections, to which (because of high mortality early in life) adaptation occurs within a few generations, the pace of human evolution is slow, and man has not adapted genetically to the changes of the last few thousand, and particularly the last few hundred, years. It is unlikely that he will adapt quickly in future, since the effectiveness of natural selection is greatly reduced in a period of low fertility and low mortality when most live-born individuals reproduce. The solution of common disease problems will not, therefore occur naturally as it did during man's evolution, by elimination of deleterious genes. It is all the more important that we should understand, and so far as possible control, environmental determinants of disease.

Against this background, the residual disease problems can be divided broadly into four classes, distinguishable according to the feasibility and means of their control. I shall refer to them as: relatively intractable; preventable, associated with poverty; preventable, associated with affluence; and potentially preventable, not known to be related to poverty or affluence.

RELATIVELY INTRACTABLE

The diseases in this class comprise the following:

(*a*) *Genetic diseases* They include the rare single-gene disorders and the more common chromosomal aberrations, most of which are eliminated as spontaneous abortions. Genetic diseases, so defined, are found in less than 0.5 per cent of live-births and, it need hardly be said, are not common diseases.

(*b*) *Other diseases determined at fertilization* These are polygenic conditions manifested mainly in late life: for example, those associated with the deterioration of the eye and the ear.

(*c*) *Diseases in which the environmental influences are prenatal* Most types of mental subnormality and of congenital malformations are in this group. The evidence, both microscopic and familial, gives no reason for thinking that such conditions are determined irreversibly at fertilization; but the influences which lead to them operate early in embryonic life, and most are likely to remain unidentified, at least in the foreseeable future.

Although the diseases in this class have in common their relative intractability, when considering the approach to them we should distinguish between abnormalities present at birth (referred to under (*a*) and (*c*)) and those manifested in late life (*b*). In the case of the serious congenital conditions such as anencephalus, Down's disease and mental subnormality, it would probably be agreed that the best solution would be the prevention of their conception or birth. But genetically determined disabilities in the elderly may come at the end of a long and healthy life, and it would be absurd to suggest that the loss at that time of vision, hearing, mobility or even sanity would make it desirable to avoid the birth of those who would be affected.

In designating these diseases as relatively intractable, I am not suggesting that they offer no scope for prevention or treatment. The withdrawal of thalidomide, the prevention of Rhesus haemolytic disease, and the treatment of phenylketonuria are notable examples, quite different in kind, of measures which have been successful in the handling of problems in this class. Nevertheless, I believe that most of them will prove to be relatively intractable, and that even in the third group ((c) above) solutions will not often arise (as in the case of the malformations caused by thalidomide or rubella) from recognition of adverse environmental influences. The significance of this conclusion for research will be considered in Chapter 12.

PREVENTABLE, ASSOCIATED WITH POVERTY

It is broadly true to say that in the past the predominant health problems – the infections – were associated with poverty, for it was the removal of influences such as malnutrition, defective hygiene and bad living and working conditions that led to their decline. However, many people in advanced countries are now largely protected from these risks, but face others related to an excess rather than a deficiency of resources. It might therefore be said that the residual problems are chiefly those associated with affluence, and that a discussion of health in the future should be focused exclusively on them.

While recognizing that the division between the transitional and industrial periods is in a sense quite arbitrary – I have merely separated the problems of the past three centuries from those of the present and foreseeable future – I think it is not possible to overlook the continuing importance of ill-health derived from poverty. In a large part of the world it is still predominant, and even in the developed countries there are people whose health needs owe more to poverty than to affluence. It is therefore necessary to assess the scope for further advances through wider application of the traditional measures: nutritional, environmental, behavioural and therapeutic.

A useful basis for this assessment is a comparison of health indices of different populations and of different sections of the same population. Table 7.1 gives the life expectation at birth for children born around 1970. The difference between the continents with the highest estimate (Europe, 71) and the lowest (Africa, 43) was nearly thirty years. Even better figures have been recorded for single countries such as Sweden (72.1 for males and 77.7 for females in 1971–2).

TABLE 7.1. *Life expectation at birth in different continents.**

Africa	43
America	65
Asia (excluding USSR)	55
Europe (excluding USSR)	71
Oceania	68
USSR	70
World total	55

* *World Health Statistics Annual*, I (1972), p. 787, WHO, Geneva.

However, when comparing developed and developing countries we must remember that most of the latter are in tropical and sub-tropical areas where there are special disease problems not seen or rarely seen in temperate zones. Hence it cannot be said that the differences are due wholly to poverty, for although health in Bangladesh or rural India could be brought much nearer to that in Scandinavia if resources were unlimited, it is unlikely that it could be raised to the same level.

This reservation does not arise in comparisons between technologically advanced countries in temperate parts of the world. Fig. 7.1 shows the trend of infant mortality (deaths of live-born children in the first year of life) in six countries between 1950 and 1975. At the beginning of this period the highest rate (in Japan) was three times the lowest (in Sweden); at the end of it the highest (in Scotland) was still nearly twice that of the lowest (again in Sweden).

A good deal can also be learned from social class differences within the same country. In Britain the population is divided for statistical purposes into five classes identified according to the occupation of the householder. Fig. 7.2 shows mortality in 1970-2 for still-births, infants under 1 year, children aged 1-14 and adults aged 15-64. The first two are expressed as death-rates (per thousand total births and per thousand live-births respectively) and the last two as standardized mortality ratios (SMRs). In all four groups there is a striking increase in mortality from the wealthiest class (I) to the poorest (V).

The class differences are greatest in relation to infective and parasitic diseases and diseases of the respiratory system, but are also quite marked for malignant neoplasms, diseases of the nervous system and sense organs, diseases of the digestive system, diseases of the genito-urinary system, and accidents, poisonings and violence.

Some of the variation in death-rates between countries and between social classes can be accounted for in other ways; for example, by deaths

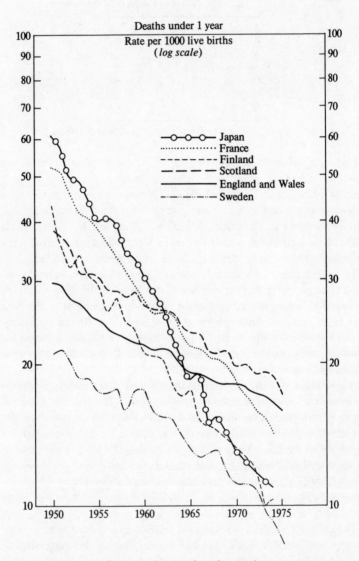

FIGURE 7.1. Infant mortality in selected countries, 1950–1975,
Source: *Prevention and death: reducing the risk*, HMSO, London, 1977, p. 13.

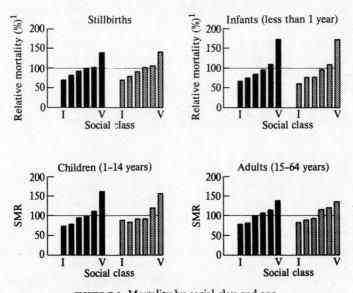

FIGURE 7.2. Mortality by social class and age

Source: *Occupational mortality, 1970–72*, HMSO, London, 1978, p. 196.

from tropical diseases in developing countries and, less certainly, by
differences in behaviour between the classes. (There is some evidence
that smoking is now more commom among the poor than among the
well-to-do, and this would increase mortality from malignant neoplasms and some other causes of death, both infective and non-infective.) However, I think there is little doubt that the differences in health
experience are attributable mainly to the direct or indirect effects of
poverty, and would be largely eliminated if it were possible to raise
the lower standards of living and medical care to the level of the highest.

PREVENTABLE, ASSOCIATED WITH AFFLUENCE

There are two lines of evidence which lead to the conclusion that disease is now often associated with affluence. One is the observation that
certain types of behaviour characteristic of an affluent society – over-
eating, physical inactivity, smoking, etc. – may cause sickness or death;
the other is the finding that some specific diseases such as cirrhosis of
the liver and cancer of the lung are attributable mainly to influences of
this kind.

Although about two-thirds of the people in the world are still under-nourished, for the first time in history there are countries where the opportunity to overeat is no longer confined to a small minority. In England and Wales young and middle-aged men are now on average about 14 lb. heavier than those of the same age and height in the 1930s, and American men are even heavier. Life insurance statistics provide impressive evidence of the effects of obesity. Men who are more than 25 per cent above the average for their age and height have a death-rate twice as high as those within 5 per cent. The differences are due to an increase in deaths from several causes, particularly ischaemic heart disease, diabetes, cerebrovascular disease, chronic nephritis and accidents.

It has also been shown that mortality from coronary artery disease increases with physical inactivity. This relationship was first demonstrated by comparison of death-rates in a wide range of occupations listed in national statistics; it has been confirmed by examination of experience of the disease among workers in occupations which differ in their physical demands: bus drivers and conductors; government clerks and postmen; long-shore men in active and less active groups. Although the mechanism by which physical activity protects from coronary artery disease is still unclear, the basic finding itself is not in doubt.

The association between cirrhosis of the liver and consumption of alcohol is even more striking, but it is well known and need not be discussed at length.

The importance of influences related to affluence, and the difficulties in some cases of establishing unequivocably their relationship to disease, are well illustrated by the present status of evidence in cancer. It varies from conclusive to suggestive.

The link between smoking and cancer of the lung is the most convincing, since it meets epidemiological requirements which might be regarded as analogous to Koch's postulates in the case of the infections.

1. There is an epidemic of the disease.
2. A plausible agent (smoking) is associated with the disease.
3. The use of the agent has increased and the increase is in the expected temporal relation to the epidemic of the disease (in both sexes).
4. Removal of the agent has lowered mortality from the disease (in doctors).

In respect of cancer of the intestine it has been suggested that the frequent occurrence in advanced countries of a condition which is rare in rural communities of developing countries may be due to the change in diet, particularly refinement of food and removal of fibre. If this explanation is correct it is understandable that two of the four lines of evidence listed above cannot be met. The refinement of food began long before cause of death was registered (in *Eugenie Grandet*, written in the 1830s, Balzac referred to the separation of the bran from the flour at the mill of the old miser); hence there are no records of the onset of the epidemic of the disease or of increased consumption of the possible causal agent (refined foods).

In the case of breast cancer, variation in frequency in different sections of the population, particularly in relation to fertility, is very suggestive of environmental influences; but again, and for obvious reasons, the evidence is deficient. Large changes in reproduction, perhaps the most profound in human history, were associated with the transition from high to low birth-rates in the past century. They have modified the age at first pregnancy, the interval between pregnancies, the age at last pregnancy and the total number of pregnancies, as well as associated practices such as intercourse, conception, and breast-feeding. It seems quite possible that one or more of these changes has been associated with an increase in prevalence of breast cancer, but if so the trends were too early to be demonstrated in national records.

Finally, there is a report of an interesting attempt to relate personal behaviour more generally to physical status. Belloc and Breslow assessed the effects on health of following seven rules which would have delighted Montaigne, an early advocate of self-discipline and moderation:[1] (*a*) don't smoke cigarettes; (*b*) sleep for seven hours; (*c*) eat breakfast; (*d*) keep weight down; (*e*) drink moderately; (*f*) exercise daily; (*g*) don't eat between meals.

The results were almost too good to be true; virtue is not often so handsomely rewarded, and indeed it is not easy to believe that seven hours of sleep and taking breakfast are equivalent as health practices to not smoking and maintaining constant weight. However, it was concluded that health and longevity increased with the number of rules followed. For people aged over 75 following all the rules, health was said to be as good as for those aged 35–44 who followed less than three; and life expectation at age 45 was 11 years longer for people following six or seven rules than for those following less than four.

1. Belloc, N. B. and Breslow, L., 'Relationship of physical health status and health practices', *Preventive Medicine*, 1 (1972), 409.

Belloc, N. B., 'Relationship of health practices and mortality', *Preventive Medicine*, 2 (1973), 67.

POTENTIALLY PREVENTABLE, NOT KNOWN TO BE RELATED
TO POVERTY OR AFFLUENCE

There remain a number of diseases which do not fit clearly into any of the preceding classes. In principle they are preventable, for there is no reason to believe they are determined irreversibly at fertilization or that the environmental influences which lead to them are prenatal. However, they have not responded to the improvements in conditions of life or advances in medicine which led to the decline of the infections; nor are they known to have arisen from changes associated with affluence.

They are a heterogeneous group. They include some acute respiratory infections, such as the common cold, influenza and viral pneumonia, as well as gastro-intestinal diseases due to viruses. More tentatively, I suggest that many psychiatric conditions are in the same class. A few of them have responded to advances in the standard of living and medical care; for example tertiary syphilis, once a frequent cause of admission to mental hospitals and, probably, diseases associated with toxic hazards and nutritional deficiencies. There are some striking differences in hospital admission rates of schizophrenics – for example between native-born and 'new' Australians (those who have recently emigrated from Europe) – which may be related to poverty. And there are remarkable instances of variation in disease experience which may be affected by affluence: the wide differences in the incidence of peptic ulcer in countries of western Europe, and the change in the male/female ratio of deaths due to perforation from peptic ulcer in New York City during this century (from one to one to about twenty to one). With such exceptions, which are not easily interpreted, there is little clear evidence that the common forms of neurotic, psychotic and psychosomatic illnesses are directly associated with either poverty or affluence.

Finally, a number of physical diseases (for example, multiple sclerosis, rheumatoid arthritis, most cases of renal disease and a minority of cancers) must be put in this heterogeneous class, often because not enough is known about their origins to enable us to judge the nature of the significant influences in their aetiology.

RESIDUAL INFLUENCES ON HEALTH

In the preceding discussion diseases were divided broadly into two categories according to the possibility of their prevention by control of environmental (non-genetic) influences. Those in the first category were considered to be relatively intractable, on the grounds that they are due to abnormalities of genes or chromosomes, or, if they are not, that the influences which lead to them are likely to be inaccessible because they are prenatal. Most of these conditions are present at birth, although some are not recognized until later (certain cases of congenital heart disease) and others are not manifested until late life. Diseases of this type can be thought of as the price to be paid for the advantages which accrue from the intricate exchange of genes at fertilization and a prolonged period of intra-uterine life. The solution of such problems depends on the prevention of their conception or birth, or on clinical intervention as in the treatment of cardiac malformations or, in late life, an arthritic hip.

By definition all other diseases are due to post-natal influences, although the feasibility of their prevention on the basis of present knowledge varies enormously. The predominant causes of ill-health in the past, infectious diseases, were determined by conditions created by the first agricultural revolution, the aggregation of populations and associated poverty, and the modern improvement in health was brought about by their removal or modification.

On a world view it might be said that the major influences on health are unchanged. In many countries in Asia, Africa and Latin America the infections are still predominant; malnutrition remains the most serious cause of disease, hygienic conditions are usually primitive and population growth is not effectively controlled. Even among the advanced countries conditions are not uniformly good, for there are considerable differences in health indices between countries and between population groups within the same country. Hence for the world as a whole the order of importance of the chief influences is probably the same as in the past – nutritional, environmental, behavioural and clinical. However, some of the variation in developed countries, for example in perinatal mortality, is now considerably affected by differences in standards of medical care.

The balance between diseases associated with poverty and those associated with affluence is changing, and there are grounds for thinking that in some advanced countries the latter are already predominant. They are determined by personal behaviour in which the changes are comparatively recent: for example, refined foods became widely available from the early nineteenth century; sedentary living dates from the introduction of mechanized transport, particularly the automobile; and cigarette smoking on a significant scale has occurred only in recent decades.

Although the relative importance of behavioural and other influences cannot be estimated accurately, it is possible to assess the ill-effects of one of them, namely smoking. Table 7.2 shows for smokers (25 cigarettes daily and over) and non-smokers of various ages, the increase in expectation of life which occurred between 1838–54 and 1970. From age 25 the increase for smokers was about half or less than half of that

TABLE 7.2. *Increase in expectation of life of males in the period 1838–54 to 1970.**

Age	Non-smokers	Smokers of 25+ CPD
0	31.9	26.0
25	13.2	7.0
35	10.3	4.1
45	7.4	2.1
55	4.6	0.6
65	2.3	0.3

* Based on mortality experience of (*a*) British doctors, smokers and non-smokers and (*b*) estimates of life expectation of males in England and Wales in 1838–54 and 1970.

for non-smokers. This result can be interpreted to mean that in the past century the improvement in expectation of life of mature males *from all causes* has been reduced by at least half by smoking alone. The fact that so large a reduction has been due to a single practice suggests that in advanced countries behavioural influences are now more important than others; and since the changes in behaviour are characteristic of an affluent society, it seems permissible to conclude that diseases associated with affluence are now predominant. The order of importance of the influences on health has altered to this extent, that personal behaviour is now relatively more significant than food deficiency and environmental hazards.

8

Medical Achievement

In Part One I concluded that the contribution of clinical medicine to the prevention of death and increase in expectation of life in the past three centuries was smaller than that of other influences. This is not of course the only index of medical achievement; doctors are also concerned largely with postponement of death (from specific causes) and treatment of non-fatal diseases, as well as with the care of patients for whom little can be done by active intervention. However, while recognizing that all these contributions are important, I think it is desirable to put them into perspective, and this can be done by considering the following question.

Let us suppose that a parent is asked to choose between two possibilities for a new-born child: that it should have the benefit of the increase in expectation of life since the beginning of the eighteenth century (from about 30 years to over 70) with the associated reduction of morbidity from the diseases that have declined, but be denied all other medical treatment; or that it should have such treatment, but return to the former high risk of death in early life, with about 30 per cent of surviving to maturity. The choice here is between the benefits that have resulted from the decline of mortality and all others not reflected in this index. No well-informed person would doubt that the parent should choose the former. This way of looking at things may seem highly theoretical, but it has a considerable bearing on health policy decisions, particularly in developing countries where a choice has to be made between investment in preventive and therapeutic measures.

However, an appraisal of all aspects of medical achievement is needed as a background for discussion of the medical role, and I shall consider it in relation to: prevention of death; postponement of death; and treatment of non-fatal diseases.

PREVENTION OF DEATH

Although the contribution of medicine under this heading has already been examined (Chapters 4 and 5), we must look at it more closely in the period when clinical procedures became effective. This is desirable not only to put the record straight, but also if we are to use medical achievement in the past as a guide to its possibilities in the future. For this purpose the last thirty years are in some respects more instructive than the previous three hundred.

TUBERCULOSIS

Mortality from tuberculosis fell sharply from the time when it was first recorded, so that a large part of the decline occurred before the introduction of effective treatment in 1947 (Fig. 8.1). However, a graph on

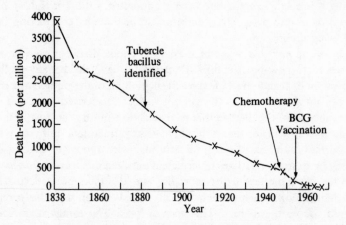

FIGURE 8.1. Respiratory tuberculosis: mean annual death-rates (standardized to 1901 population): England and Wales.

this scale conceals the large contribution made by chemotherapy in the later stages, so we need to examine the death-rate more closely immediately before and after streptomycin came into use. Since experience of the disease varies by age and sex, death-rates since 1921 are shown separately for males and females in three age groups: under 15; 15–44; and 45 and over (Figs. 8.2 and 8.3). Straight lines have been fitted to

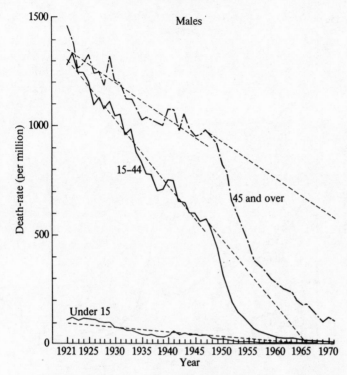

FIGURE 8.2. Respiratory tuberculosis: annual death-rates of males: England and Wales.

the rates for the years 1921 to 1946, and extrapolated to 1971, allowing for the slight increase between 1946 and 1947.

On the assumption that without streptomycin the decline of mortality would have continued at about the same rate as between 1921 and 1946, estimates have been made of the contribution of treatment. The results are given in Table 8.1, for the sexes combined. Chemotherapy reduced the number of deaths in the period since it was introduced (1948–71) by 51 per cent; for the whole period since cause of death was first recorded (1848–71) the reduction was 3.2 per cent.

BCG vaccination was used from about the same time as streptomycin and it is therefore difficult to separate the effects of the two measures. In the examination of the trend of mortality (Table 8.1) it was assumed that the benefit was due wholly to chemotherapy. That this assumption is not unreasonable is suggested by the experience of the Netherlands,

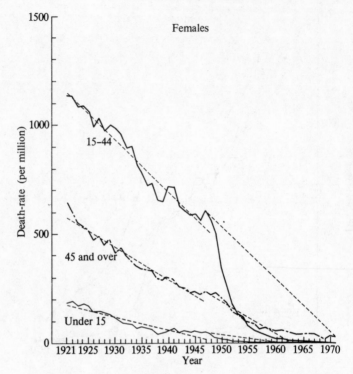

FIGURE 8.3. Respiratory tuberculosis: annual death-rates of females:
England and Wales.

TABLE 8.1. *Estimated number of deaths from respiratory tuberculosis
prevented by use of chemotherapy: England and Wales.*

	1948–1971	1848–1971
Estimated by extrapolation*	273,727	4,377,265
Actual	133,891	4,237,429
Deaths prevented	139,836	139,836
Proportion of deaths prevented	51%	3.2%

* Of 1921–46 rates.

which has never had a national BCG programme, but nevertheless had
the lowest death-rates from respiratory tuberculosis for any European
country in 1957–9 and 1967–9 (Fig. 8.4).

The history of tuberculosis illustrates, perhaps better than that of any
other infection, a general point about the contribution of therapy.

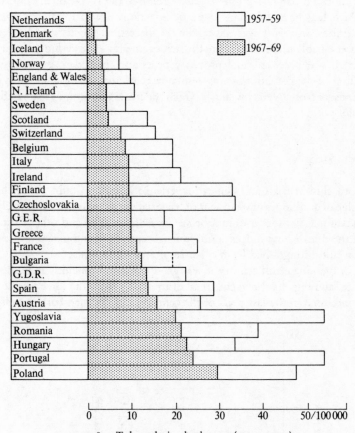

Deaths from Tuberculosis
(per 100,000)

FIGURE 8.4. Tuberculosis: death-rates (per 100,000).

Sources: *World Health Statistics Report*, **23**, no. 8 (1970);
World Health Statistics Annual, **1** (1970).

Effective clinical intervention came late in the history of the disease, and over the whole period of its decline the effect was small in relation to that of other influences. But although the problems presented by tuberculosis in the mid twentieth century were smaller than those in the early nineteenth, it was still a common and often fatal disease with a high level of associated morbidity. In two of its forms, tuberculous meningitis and miliary tuberculosis, it was invariably fatal. The challenge to medical science and practice was to increase the rate of decline of mortality, and, if possible, finally remove the threat of the disease which had been a leading cause of infectious deaths for nearly two centuries. In this it was outstandingly successful, and it would be as unreasonable to underestimate this achievement as to overlook the fact that it was preceded, and probably necessarily preceded, by modification of the conditions – low resistance from malnutrition and heavy exposure from overcrowding – which had made tuberculosis so formidable.

PNEUMONIA

Both clinical trials and clinical experience leave no doubt about the value of antibiotics in treatment of bacterial pneumonia. Unfortunately in national statistics it cannot be separated from viral and other forms of the disease, and indeed, until quite recently, pneumonia (all causes) was not distinguished from other respiratory infections.

In the nineteenth century it was grouped with bronchitis and influenza, and Fig. 8.5 shows the trend of mortality from the three diseases. It increased in the last years of the century, but declined fairly rapidly

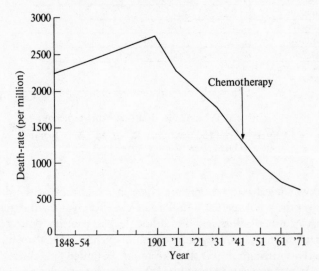

FIGURE 8.5. Bronchitis, pneumonia, and influenza: death-rates (standardized to 1901 population): England and Wales.

from about 1900. It is hardly surprising that there is no visible change in the slope of the curve after the introduction of chemotherapy, since the diagram is based mainly on conditions in which antibiotics are not effective.

For England and Wales it is possible to examine the death-rate from pneumonia (all causes) from 1931, and Figs. 8.6 and 8.7 show the rates for males and females respectively in three age groups. Mortality fell during the whole period, and at ages 0–14 and 45–64 the rate of decline

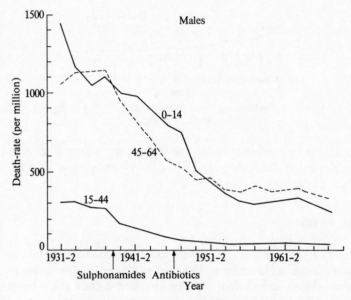

FIGURE 8.6. Pneumonia: mean annual death-rates of males: England and Wales.

increased after the use of sulphonamides and antibiotics; there was little difference in the 15–44 age group. In the same period deaths from pneumonia rose sharply for both sexes at ages over 65, but here interpretation is even more difficult since the many different causes of death included under this heading in old people make the diagnosis wholly unreliable.

These data cast no doubt on the effectiveness of antibiotics in the treatment of bacterial pneumonia. What they do show is that mortality from respiratory diseases certified initially under 'bronchitis, influenza

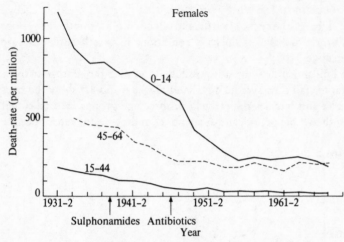

FIGURE 8.7. Pneumonia: mean annual death-rates of females:
England and Wales.

and pneumonia', and later under pneumonia, was falling from about
the beginning of the century, and that its continued decline after 1935
was not due mainly to chemotherapy.

DIPHTHERIA

Mortality from diphtheria in England and Wales has fallen fairly continuously since the late nineteenth century (Fig. 8.8), when treatment
by antitoxin was introduced. The rate increased slightly at the beginning of the last war, but fell rapidly from about the time when a national
programme of immunization began. Diphtheria is now a rare disease,
and many doctors trained since the Second World War have never seen
it. In the six years from 1965 to 1970, there were only nine deaths from
diphtheria in England and Wales.

It is tempting to attribute the decline of diphtheria deaths between
1895 and 1922 to treatment by antitoxin, and the rapid fall since 1940
to immunization. Nothing in the evidence is seriously inconsistent with
this interpretation, and if mortality from the other common infections
had increased or remained constant in the same period it could possibly
be accepted unreservedly. But the fact that, without prophylaxis or
treatment, diseases such as whooping cough and measles also caused
far fewer deaths, suggests that other influences may also have been at

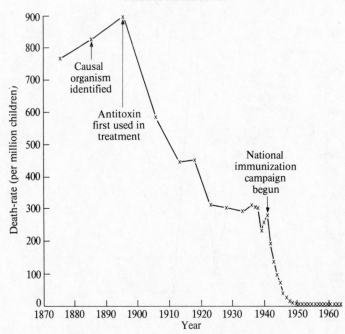

FIGURE 8.8. Diphtheria: death rates of children under 15:
England and Wales.

work in diphtheria. With due regard for this reservation it seems probable that immunization had more effect on the control of this disease than of any other, with the exceptions of poliomyelitis and, possibly, smallpox. This conclusion is supported by the high level of immunity which follows the use of a good antigen. Evidence for England and Wales in 1961–3 indicated that the risk of an attack of diphtheria was about six times greater, and the risk of a fatal attack ten times greater, in those not immunized than in those immunized.

SMALLPOX

Fig. 8.9 shows the trend of mortality from smallpox in England and Wales since cause of death was first registered. Unfortunately, there are no reliable data for the eighteenth and earlier centuries, but the London Bills of Mortality suggest that epidemics of the disease caused many deaths, particularly among children. In 1796 one-fifth of all deaths in

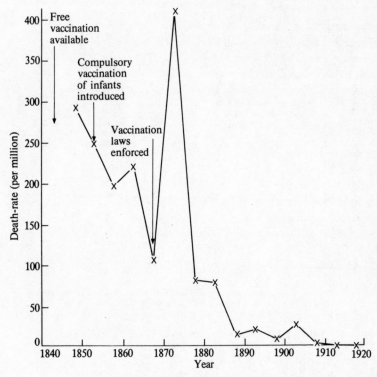

FIGURE 8.9. Smallpox: death rates: England and Wales.

London were ascribed to smallpox. Mortality declined rapidly from the late nineteenth century and since about 1910 there have been relatively few deaths in the British Isles.

Vaccination was used first in 1798, made compulsory in 1852, and enforced rigorously between 1872 and 1887, when the acceptance rate for children was about 90 per cent. But parents increasingly took advantage of the concientious objection clause, and in 1948, when compulsion ceased, less than 40 per cent of infants were vaccinated. In 1971 it was decided that vaccination should no longer be recommended as a routine procedure in early childhood.

It is not easy to assess accurately the contribution that vaccination has made to the decline of mortality from smallpox. Creighton, the historian of infectious disease, considered it useless; but this view is generally regarded as perverse and inconsistent with the evidence. In the light of present knowledge of the high degree of protection afforded by vaccination for a limited period it seems reasonable to believe that the procedure was very effective in the late nineteenth century when a high proportion of children were immunized, and still more in the measures taken more recently to prevent the spread of the disease by identification and vaccination of people exposed to smallpox.

POLIOMYELITIS

Poliomyelitis appears to have been a rare disease before the late nineteenth century, but since that time it has occurred in epidemics in many countries. The number of people infected but with few or no clinical manifestations exceeds greatly (by about 100 to one) the number affected by paralysis.

Because of the crippling disabilities which are common in patients

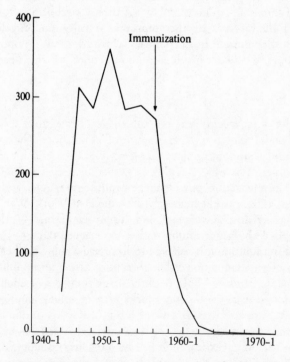

FIGURE 8.10. Poliomyelitis: mean annual notification rates of children under 15: England and Wales.

who survive, there is some tendency to overestimate the importance of poliomyelitis in relation to other infections. In 1947, when the highest death-rate was recorded in England and Wales, there were 33 deaths per million children under 15, compared with 99 from whooping cough and 69 from measles. In 1871–80, before the decline in mortality began, the last two diseases were responsible for 1415 and 1038 deaths (per million under 15) respectively.

Since the number of deaths from poliomyelitis is small, the reduction in mortality made little contribution to the decline of the overall death-rate. However, the disabling effects are so serious that the trend of notifications is more important than in other infections.

This is shown in Fig. 8.10 for England and Wales. The rate fell sharply from 1956 when immunization was introduced, and by 1964–5 there were few cases. This strongly suggests that immunization was responsible for the reduction of notifications and prevention of disabilities and deaths. Moreover, laboratory evidence indicates that it gives a high degree of immunity, as measured by the titre of circulating antibodies. Results of clinical trials are also impressive. Finally, poliomyelitis has been almost eliminated from countries which have had immunization programmes, whereas it is still common in countries which have not.

TETANUS

Before the First World War the annual death-rate from tetanus in England and Wales was 7 per million of population. The rate has fallen almost continuously since that time (Fig. 8.11) and is now well below 0.5 per million.

Passive immunization, in which tetanus antitoxin is given at the time of injury, has been used extensively since the First World War. However, it has certain disadvantages, and during the Second World War it was replaced by active immunization by tetanus toxoid.

Passive immunization is believed to have had a substantial effect on mortality from tetanus, and although routine active immunization of children was introduced only recently, large numbers of adults have been protected since the Second World War, including all those who served in the armed forces. But while it is probable that immunization contributed substantially, other explanations (such as the disappearance of the horse from the roads) must be found for the considerable reduction of deaths before it was used. It should also be mentioned that in recent years there has been a significant improvement in treatment.

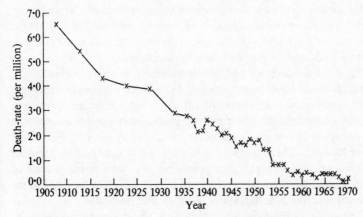

FIGURE 8.11. Tetanus: mean annual death rates: England and Wales.

WHOOPING COUGH

The death-rate from whooping cough in England and Wales (Fig. 8.12) has declined since the seventh decade of the nineteenth century. The effectiveness of treatment is still in doubt, and the more important issue is the contribution of immunization.

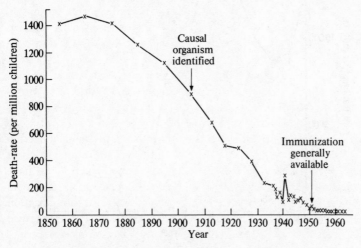

FIGURE 8.12. Whooping cough: death rates of children under 15: England and Wales.

As mortality had fallen to a low level before immunization was introduced, its value must be judged in relation to morbidity, of which the evidence is the trend of notifications. This source is notoriously unsatisfactory, because frequently cases are not notified.

The rate has declined almost continuously since 1950 (Fig. 8.13), although there have been periodic, by former experience relatively small, epidemics. Unfortunately for the purposes of interpretation, immunization tends to be introduced gradually and it is not easy to be certain when it was first used extensively. The Annual Report of the Chief Medical Office suggests that the procedure may not have been in general use until at least a few years after the onset of the decline of notifications. It has also been observed that in Germany, where immunization was not used nationally, notifications decreased.

Opinion, including medical opinion, is still divided over the relative advantages and disadvantages of immunization against whooping cough. A decision is important in practice; but it is not essential for this

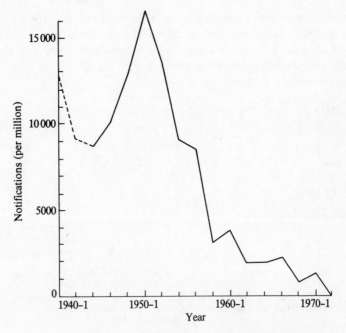

FIGURE 8.13. Whooping cough: mean annual notification rates of children under 15: England and Wales.

analysis, and in concluding that the matter is still open I recall Haldane's remark, that in a scientific paper one can almost gauge the intellectual honesty of the author by the number of phenomena he or she leaves unexplained'.[1]

MEASLES

With some variation in timing, the history of measles has been rather similar to that of whooping cough. The death-rate fell continuously from about 1915 (Fig. 8.14); treatment (of secondary infections) has been possible since 1935; and mortality was at a low level before immunization was used.

Fig. 8.15 shows the trend of notifications. The rate decreased from 1950 to 1956, was more or less constant to 1960, and declined rapidly

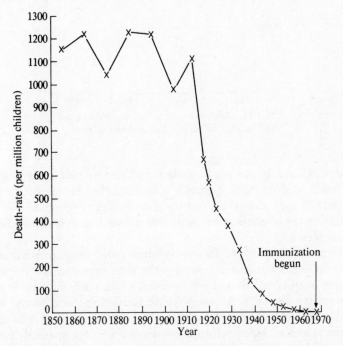

FIGURE 8.14. Measles: death rates of children under 15: England and Wales.

1. Haldane, J. B. S., *Science and Life* (London: Pemberton, 1968), p. 65.

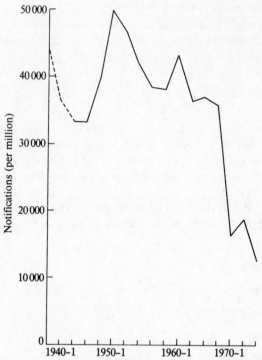

FIGURE 8.15. Measles: mean annual notification rates.
of children under 15: England and Wales.

after that time. It was not until mid 1968 that vaccination was used nationally and less than a quarter of all children had been protected by the end of 1972. I conclude that the contribution of immunization to the reduction of notifications in the last decade cannot be decided on this evidence.

There are many other infections in which prophylaxis and treatment are effective. Internationally perhaps the most important are tropical diseases such as malaria and yellow fever, which really fall outside the scope of this discussion. Although syphilis had declined for other reasons, it was still important when salvarsan became available early in this century, and mortality fell to a low level before the arsenicals were replaced by penicillin. Other treatable infectious diseases include bacterial meningitis, sub-acute bacterial endocarditis, typhoid, osteo-myelitis, puerperal fever, bacterial infections of the ear, pharynx and larynx, cellulitis, gonorrhoea, carbuncle and cystitis. Some of these conditions are usually fatal if untreated; others are important as causes of morbidity rather than mortality.

This appraisal of some of the most important medical advances leaves little doubt that their impact was much smaller than is generally believed. The infections were declining long before successful intervention was possible, and since that time, with some notable exceptions (especially in the case of tuberculosis and poliomyelitis) immunization and treatment were less effective than other influences. It is significant that some procedures which were carefully assessed by randomized control trials (for example BCG vaccination) do not appear to have had the expected results. The conclusion which seems inescapable is that the influences which determine man's response to infectious disease–genetic, nutritional, environmental and behavioural, as well as medical–are infinitely complex, and we need to be very cautious before assuming that we fully understand the infections, or that we have in our hands the certain means of their control.

NON-INFECTIVE CONDITIONS

The chief requirement for an understanding of health in the past is an explanation of the rise and fall of infectious diseases. In relation to the future, however, assessment of achievements with non-communicable diseases is, arguably, more significant. In developed countries, they are now the predominant causes of sickness and death, and what has been achieved in the understanding and control of such conditions is therefore a valuable, if incomplete, indication of future possibilities.

Unfortunately it is very difficult to assess the achievements. In the first place, because non-communicable diseases vary greatly in severity, duration and the extent of associated morbidity and disability, mortality is a far less satisfactory index than in the case of the infections, where the outcome is often either death or complete recovery. Secondly, many clinical procedures have never been satisfactorily evaluated, and their use is based on indirect laboratory evidence or on clinical impressions. A short assessment of the medical contribution can therefore be little more than a list of conditions in which clinical intervention is generally believed to be effective.

In his thoughtful examination of medical advances in the period 1950–75, after discussing the management of infectious diseases Thomas concluded that the list of decisive new accomplishments is not much longer than the contents of the following paragraph.

There have been a few other examples of technology improvement, comparable in decisive effectiveness, since 1950, but the best of these have been for relatively uncommon illnesses. Childhood leukemia and certain solid tumors in children, for example, can now be cured by chemotherapy in a substantial proportion of cases, but there are only a few thousand of these per year in the country. Endocrine-replacement therapy has become highly effective and relatively inexpensive ('relative' considering the cost of caring for untreated endocrine abnormalities) for a variety of disorders involving the adrenals, pituitary, parathyroid, ovary, and thyroid; in particular, the biochemical treatment of thyroid dysfunction has improved markedly. Hematology has offered new and effective replacement treatment for certain anemias. Immunological prophylaxis now prevents most cases of hemolytic disease of the newborn. Progress in anesthesia, electrolyte physiology, and cardiopulmonary physiology has greatly advanced the field of surgery, so that reparative and other procedures can now be done which formerly were technically impossible.[2]

This paragraph provides a reasonable summary of decisive advances, some of which were launched before 1950. To them should be added the treatment of malignant hypertension and, in some cases, essential hypertension. Successful measures also include the treatment of accidents, surgical treatment of cardiac conditions, relief of prostatic obstruction, renal transplants and cure of a minority of cancers. Treatment of obstetric conditions may be life-saving, as the valuable investigations of maternal mortality in Britain have shown. So too is intervention in other emergencies (abdominal obstruction, perforated peptic ulcer). There are many therapies (referred to below) which postpone rather than prevent death from a specific cause, or provide relief of symptoms without affecting expectation of life, which in many disorders is not threatened.

What should be noted about these advances is that they are not restricted to preventable disorders, such as accidents, which in an ideal world would not occur. They include conditions classified in the preceding chapter as relatively intractable. The prevention of rhesus haemolytic disease is a remarkable example of an advance made possible by a combination of genetic and clinical knowledge. The identification and abortion of a foetus affected by Down's disease is another solution of an apparently intractable problem made possible by application of

2. Thomas, L., 'On the science and technology of medicine' in *Daedalus* (Winter, 1977), p. 37.

genetic knowledge. Equally impressive in a quite different way is the immense technical accomplishment which restores a child with a patent ductus arteriosus or an atrial septal defect to a life of normal duration and quality. Such achievements suggest that further investigation may make it possible to prevent, eliminate or treat successfully some of the most difficult disorders with which medicine is now confronted.

POSTPONEMENT OF DEATH

The use of the decline of mortality as the main index of improvement in health is sometimes said to overlook the contribution of medical intervention which postpones death but does not change its cause. Diabetes is cited as an example of a disease in which the extension of life is not reflected in the trend of mortality, because the same cause often appears later on a death certificate.

The interpretation of death-rates is admittedly complex. They are based on the number dying (the numerator) over the total population (the denominator). If deaths from a disease are reduced, the death-rate from that disease and the death-rate from all causes (assuming no other changes have occurred) both fall, because the numerator is smaller and the denominator larger. This is true whether the cause of death is eliminated (as in typhoid) or postponed (as in diabetes). Moreover, in both cases the rates are permanently lowered, because the number dying in a year remains smaller in relation to the population at risk. Hence the postponement and prevention of death from a specific cause are both reflected in the index.

When examining the trend of mortality over a considerable period it is important to standardize for age changes in the population (an approximation to the ideal bases for examination, the age-specific mortality rates). The need for this procedure is evident from a comparison of death-rates from diabetes before and after insulin. In England and Wales the crude rates were 107 (per million) in 1911–20 and 125 in 1973, which would seem to imply that mortality increased over this period. When standardized to the 1973 population, the death-rate in 1911–20 was 188.

However, standardization does not remove all the difficulties of interpretation. Diabetes appears to be more common than in the past, but it is not possible to dissociate the effects of improved survival, better diagnosis and possibly other influences. Survival of diabetics has been gravely prejudiced by the increased frequency of smoking during the period when effective treatment (by insulin and oral diabetic drugs) has been available. And finally, mortality statistics are very unreliable, because many diabetics die from arterial degeneration and their deaths are often attributed to disease of the kidneys, heart and brain.

With due regard for these difficulties, useful evidence of the effect of treatment can be obtained from examination of age of death of diabetics. Fig. 8.16 shows (for England and Wales) the number of survivors of cohorts of 1,000 females exposed to the mortality rates of 1911–20 and 1973. The difference in mean age at death at the two periods was approximately ten years.

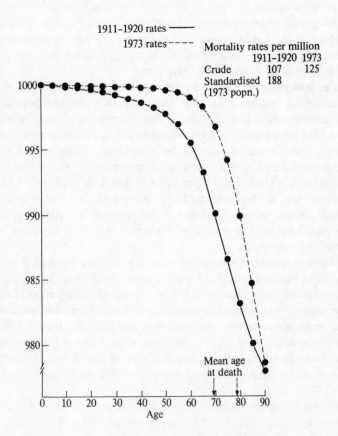

FIGURE 8.16. Survivors from a cohort of 1000 females exposed only to mortality from diabetes at rates of 1911–20 and 1973.

It may seem surprising that age at death was so late – nearly 70 in 1911–20 and nearly 80 in 1973. This is explained partly by the fact that even before insulin most diabetics died relatively late in life. (The age at death in 1911–20, and the extension of life which has resulted from treatment, would of course be vastly different if attention were restricted to juvenile diabetics.) But the late age of death is also determined by the fact that deaths of diabetics from all causes other than diabetes were inevitably excluded from the cohort, and those dying from a single cause, diabetes or any other, are highly and favourably selected in respect of length of life. This is merely another way of saying that the risk of death from a single disease already manifested is often less than the risk of death from all other causes taken together. Indeed, it could be said to many people by way of reassurance: you will be fortunate if you live long enough to die from the disease which most you fear.

For assessment of the effect of postponement of death from a single disease whose contribution to the total decline of mortality is small, the change in age-specific death-rates and increase in expectation of life are probably the best indices. But in assessment of the contribution of a large number of causes (as in the case of the non-infective conditions considered in Chapter 3), both the prevention and the postponement of death are reflected fairly accurately in the trend of the age-standardized mortality rates.

TREATMENT OF NON-FATAL DISEASES

When presenting the results of his experiments on himself a distinguished biologist seemed to say: Take one average human being, for example, J. B. S. Haldane. Adopting the same unconventional statistical approach, we can illustrate the relation between morbidity and mortality by considering the experience of one lakeland poet. William Wordsworth followed most of the rules for health now advocated by life stylists. He did not smoke or drink; unlike some of his best friends he avoided opium; he lived and worked in the open air, added little weight and took an amount of exercise which would have daunted most joggers. De Quincey estimated that Wordsworth walked between 175,000 and 180,000 miles during his life, and if so he must have averaged nearly ten miles a day for sixty years.

Predictably, according to the health rules, he had a long life. However, he and his sister both suffered a good deal from minor morbidity – headaches, toothaches, bowel upsets and numerous other unspecified complaints – recorded meticulously by Dorothy in her *Journals* during their years in Dove Cottage. As for his mental health, it has been suggested that he had an abnormal relationship with his sister, but although many of her references to him are highly suggestive, there is no evidence that it was ever consummated. What Wordsworth's history illustrates is that there is no necessary close relation between morbidity and mortality. The diseases that shorten our lives are not usually the ones that diminish their quality from day to day.

Nevertheless, there has been a large reduction in sickness associated with causes of death that have declined. This is particularly true of the chronic respiratory and venereal infections. Their contribution to the reduction of morbidity cannot be measured, but it is possible that it was greater than that from non-fatal diseases. It seems quite likely that the virtual elimination of chronic respiratory tuberculosis was the greatest single influence on declining sickness rates.

In the present context, however, we are concerned with medical achievement through treatment of diseases and disabilities that do not kill. In this assessment account must be taken of both the frequency and the seriousness of a condition: the common cold affects most people fairly frequently; rheumatoid arthritis and schizophrenia are much less common but far more disabling for those who are afflicted.

With one notable exception, there is no wholly effective treatment for the non-fatal illnesses which trouble most people from day to day. These are the acute respiratory infections, digestive disorders, the skeletal and muscular disabilities referred to as rheumatism, and a variety of mental illnesses, particularly the neuroses and psychoneuroses. The exception is dental disease. As the history of many famous people illustrates, dental diseases were formerly among the most common causes of serious discomfort; today they can be prevented and treated, and in the 1949 Survey of Sickness in Britain they accounted for only four per cent of the illnesses of which people complained most frequently. It would be interesting to have an estimate of their frequency in the past, say in the age of Pericles or the court of Louis XIV. Louis himself suffered grievously from his teeth, and no doubt would gladly have exchanged his painters, dramatists, one or two mistresses and several Peers of France for a modern dentist.

Of course a good deal can be done to relieve discomfort from the common complaints; it might also be said that many, although by no means all of them, are transient and present no permanent threat to the quality or duration of life. Nevertheless, such conditions are responsible for a great deal of ill-health, and their prevention or treatment is a legitimate goal of medical research and practice. Indeed, considering the frequency of the common cold, in the celestial counting-house where such imponderables can be weighed, its elimination might be considered as important as the treatment of one of the more serious but less prevalent diseases. Happily, only those disposing of research funds are required to make such value judgements.

There have been advances in treatment of many uncomfortable and, in some cases, disabling conditions, including hernias, piles, varicose veins, Parkinson's disease, pemphigus and ulcerative colitis. Although neither rheumatoid arthritis nor osteoarthritis can be cured, symptomatic relief can be provided and surgical treatment is sometimes remarkably successful, particularly by replacement of the diseased hip, one of the outstanding achievements of contemporary medicine. The major psychoses, schizophrenia and manic depression, are still unexplained, but drug therapy has benefited many patients and, by making them more manageable, has reduced the difficulties involved in their care. There has been little advance in the treatment of mentally subnormal patients, although they can be assisted by educational and occupational opportunities as well as personal care.

Because the non-fatal diseases vary greatly in frequency, duration and severity, it is not easy to summarize achievements in their treatment. It is a recognition of the difficulties they present rather than a criticism of medical research and practice to say that while symptomatic relief can be provided for some, perhaps all patients, with some notable exceptions the underlying conditions cannot at present be cured. This is true of the relatively benign conditions which trouble most people from day to day, and of the less common causes of serious disease and disability.

Part Three
The Role of Medicine

9

Non-Personal Health Services

In Part One the determinants of health were assessed in two ways: by examining conceptually the role of heredity and environment in the aetiology of disease (Chapter 2); and by appraisal of influences on health which have operated in the past and, having regard to the change in disease problems, can be expected to operate in future (Chapters 3–8). The conclusions derived from these different approaches are broadly consistent.

1. Most diseases, including the common ones, are not inevitable. They result from environmental influences on genetic material which is varied, complex, and, at present, little understood. In relation to the feasibility of preventing common diseases, the important issue is neither the understanding of genetic mechanisms nor the balance sheet of nature and nurture, which in any case cannot be quantified accurately; it is the practicability of controlling the environmental component. The most significant distinction is between prenatal influences, which are relatively intractable, and post-natal influences, many of which can be modified or removed.

2. This theoretical interpretation is in accord with past experience. The improvement in health since the eighteenth century was in respect of post-natal rather than prenatal conditions, and was associated predominantly with the infections, the diseases most susceptible to control. The influences which led to their predominance from the time of the first Agricultural Revolution 10,000 years ago were insufficient food, environmental hazards, and excessive numbers, and the measures which led to their decline from the time of the modern Agricultural and Industrial Revolutions were predictably improved nutrition, better hygiene, and contraception. These advances preceded effective medical intervention in the form of immunization and therapy which has made a much smaller contribution to the reduction of mortality and morbidity associated with infectious diseases.

3. The change in the character of health problems which followed the decline of the infections in developed countries has not invalidated the conclusion that most diseases, both physical and mental, are associated with influences which in principle might be controlled. But relatively more of these influences are now prenatal, and among post-natal influences those which the individual determines by his own behaviour (smoking, eating, exercise, and the like) are more important than those which depend mainly on action by society: provision of essential food and protection from hazards. The contribution to be expected from personal medical measures to the prevention of sickness and premature death remains tertiary, in relation to the predominant behavioural and environmental influences.

The disposal of society's investment in health is based on quite different premises. It is assumed that we are ill and are made well, whereas it is nearer the truth to say that we are well and are made ill. Few people think of themselves as having a major responsibility for their own health, and the enormous resources which technologically advanced countries assign to the health field are used mainly to treat disease or, to a lesser extent, to prevent it by personal measures such as immunization.

The conclusion that the predominant influences are quite different from those that have hitherto been assumed clearly has implications for health services. However, before examining them I should comment on the time likely to be required to bring about adjustments. In consideration of health services there is a tendency to think on too small a time-scale, and this is particularly evident in the United States where it is often difficult to interest planners in any proposal unlikely to appeal to Congress within the next eighteen months, less if the Administration is about to change. It should be remembered that in most advanced countries the contempory pattern of health services had its origins in the hospitals built in the eighteenth century, and is based on concepts established much earlier. We can hardly be surprised if some decades are required to modify an approach which has developed over hundreds of years.

Furthermore, a different concept of the basis of human health should not be thought of as a recipe for action whose validity is to be judged by whether it provides an immediate solution to some of the most complex problems facing society: for example, in developing countries limitation of numbers and provision of food, and in developed countries modification of behaviour and a fresh approach to personal health services based on recognition of the limited scope for therapeutic intervention and the predominance of the need for care. The enlarged understanding of health and disease should rather be regarded as a conceptual base, whose implications for services, education, and research will need to be developed progressively over a considerable period. It is therefore only a very preliminary examination of these matters which can be attempted in this chapter and those that follow.

NUTRITION

I shall begin with nutrition, which internationally is probably still the most important determinant of health. The grounds on which lack of food is regarded as the main influence in developing countries today and in all countries in the recent past were summarized in Chapters 6 and 7.

For developing countries of Asia, Africa, and Latin America, the conclusion concerning nutrition is in accord with so much recent experience that it is unnecessary to dwell at length on its implications. It is well recognized that it is essential to increase food supplies, and since they cannot be expanded very rapidly or indefinitely it is also necessary to restrict numbers. This of course was Malthus's central idea, or, perhaps more accurately, the deduction which follows from it, outlined in the opening chapter of his *Essay on Population* and stated succinctly on its first page: 'The tendency of all animated life is to increase beyond the nourishment provided for it.' The reception of this idea was coloured by reaction to the religious, social, and political opinions with which he associated it, and by well-founded doubts about the validity of his conclusion that food supplies increase arithmetically whereas populations tend to increase geometrically. The fact remains that Malthus associated the two basic notions of food deficiency and excessive numbers, and it is most unfortunate that subsequently they became dissociated in concept and practice, largely because of religious taboos on contraception. Happily the objections are being gradually withdrawn, and international organizations are at last permitted to include family planning among their aims. It should be linked so far as possible to food policies, and the related issues of improved nutrition and limitation of population growth should be given the priority they merit on the grounds that they are not only of general importance to man's welfare, but are also the major determinants of health.

The significance of food in developed countries is of course somewhat different. There it can be assumed that most people have enough to eat, and the more usual problem is consumption of excessive or ill-balanced diets. Since this is determined by personal choice as well as by custom and public policy, it should be regarded as a behavioural influence on health. However, even in the wealthiest countries there are sections of the population which are still inadequately, as distinct from unwisely, fed. In proportion and composition they probably vary from one country to another, but in developed countries they are mainly in two classes, the late children of large families and elderly people, particularly those living alone.

There is of course general concern about the welfare of such groups, and in Britain efforts are made to assist them, for example by family allowances, Home Helps, and Meals-on-Wheels. Nevertheless they do not have the attention they would be given if it were recognized that food is critical to their health. Nor do they receive the kind of assistance that would be most useful, for example food supplements and subsidies such as were provided during the Second World War, and whose effectiveness was reflected in health indices in spite of deterioration in some other features of working and living conditions. If a choice must be made, free school meals are more important for the health of poor children than immunization programmes, and both are more effective than hospital beds.

The potential significance of food subsidies to health is still unrecognized. They were introduced under the exigencies of the war period as a device for restricting the cost of living, and it is hardly noticed that society has stumbled on to an efficient instrument for the promotion of health. Indeed it is often assumed that in an affluent society cheap food may be positively harmful ('Beyond a certain point more and better food appears to mean increased need for medical services'[1]) and there are some grounds for this conclusion under present economic policies which take little or no account of their impact on health. We subsidize sugar which is harmful, and make butter which contains saturated fats competitive in price with the more innocuous margarine. The cost of refined flour, remarkably, is lower than that of whole meal, and the health conscious individual who seeks to restore the fibre to his diet by the addition of bran will find that this simple commodity, which was cheap so long as it was fed only to pets and livestock, has become expensive since it was shown to be of value to man.

1. Galbraith, J. K., *The Affluent Society* (Penguin Books, 1969), p. 209.

Having regard for the importance of food to health, the aim of public policy should be to use supplements and subsidies discriminately to put essential constituents within the reach of everyone, and to provide inducements for people to prefer foods that are beneficial to those that are harmful. Of course these aims cannot be expected to exclude all other considerations, such as international agreements and the solvency of farmers who have been encouraged to produce livestock and dairy products rather than grains. Nevertheless in all future evaluations of agricultural and related economic policies, the health implications should be given a primary place.

ENVIRONMENT

In their contribution to health in the past, the hygienic measures introduced progressively from the second half of the nineteenth century were second only to nutrition. However, many well-recognized risks associated with housing, atmosphere, traffic, insect vectors and working conditions are far from being eliminated, while others inherent in contemporary life have not been fully assessed or, in some cases, recognized. In developing countries effective control of the environment has scarcely begun. In 1970 the World Health Organization reported that only 14 per cent of rural populations in the Third World had access to safe drinking water and only 8 per cent had adequate arrangements for disposal of sewage.

Public responsibility for health services was introduced in the nineteenth century primarily for the purpose of dealing with infectious diseases, and the measures initially taken were control of the physical environment and provision of services, including hospitals, for infectious patients. The new service, based on local authorities was preventive in outlook and emphasized improvements in the environment as a means of promoting health. This viewpoint was reflected in the concept of the role of the medical officer of health who was conceived by Chadwick as 'a district medical officer independent of private practice and with the securities of special qualifications and responsibilities to initiate sanitary measures'. Duncan, the first medical officer of health (in Liverpool) was 'most intimately acquainted with the sanitary conditions of which he spoke and had long given intelligent and humane consideration to means of improving them'.[2]

2. Simon, John, *English Sanitary Institutions* (London: Smith Elder and Co., 1897), p. 247.

In the present century the health work of local authorities in Britain was greatly extended, by development of personal health services (from 1906), by responsibility for public hospitals (from 1929 to 1948) and by duties related to the care and after care of the sick imposed by the National Health Service in 1948. But this extension did not remove their resposibility for environmental medicine; nor did it diminish their interest in the prevention of disease and promotion of health. The conspicuous disadvantage of traditional public health was its isolation from therapeutic services, provided since 1948 almost exclusively by other public authorities.

The 1974 reorganization eliminated this anomaly, but in unifying administration of personal medical services under the new regional and area authorities it separated them from environmental services which remain under local government. The medical specialist in environmental medicine now has a consultative rather than an executive role, and the specialist in community medicine, the heir to the public health tradition, is concerned largely with personal medical care. In such circumstances it seems important to ask whether environmental measures will receive the attention they deserve, and, more broadly, whether the new service will give due emphasis to the prevention of disease and promotion of health. Will the specialist in community medicine bring to the new administration the goals and outlook which characterized public health from its introduction in the nineteenth century? Or will the pressures of therapeutic services obscure these aims, until with a new generation of doctors who have never worked in public health they are finally forgotten?

The attitude of medicine to the environment has always been somewhat equivocal, and the first Chief Scientist probably expressed the view of most educators when he wrote: 'the most characteristic function of a doctor lies in the diagnosis and treatment of disease in the individual patient' and 'the great majority of doctors will remain concerned with disease and not with "positive health" or "community medicine" or "social medicine" '.[3] This viewpoint is reflected in medical education, which gives little attention to environmental influences and measures needed for their control.

This approach might have been accepted, with reservations, when a special class of doctors was responsible for the prevention of disease and

3. Black, D. A. K., *The Logic of Medicine* (Edinburgh and London: Oliver and Boyd, 1968).

the promotion of health. But the specialist in community medicine is now concerned largely with personal health services, and it cannot be taken for granted that he will have the same influence on environmental medicine as his predecessor in public health. However, it might be argued that such a change would not be serious, since the measures needed to improve the environment are already largely in the hands of non-medical people.

It is not easy for doctors to accept that medicine is not vitally concerned with the major determinants of health. However, this reaction might be dismissed as professional chauvinism if there were no more tangible grounds for thinking that it is important to retain, and indeed to extend medical interest in investigation and control of hazards. These grounds are as follows.

In spite of improvements the environment still presents many and varied threats to health. They are more complex than in the past; for example, it was easier to recognize, measure, and control the risks of infected water and polluted air than those associated with drug therapy and radiological examination of the breast. Moreover, in a highly industrialized society, the risks are constantly changing.

Responsibility is already very fragmented, different administrations being concerned with measures related to: (a) occupation; (b) local matters such as housing, water supplies, and atmospheric pollution; (c) national issues such as air, rail, and road travel and pollution of sea and rivers; and (d) risks arising from medical investigation and treatment. The work associated with such large and complex problems must of course involve many administrations and professions, but it seems inevitable that there will be serious omissions so long as there is no organization, local as well as central, with a more comprehensive responsibility for surveillance.

It also seems essential to have a medical contribution. The scope of inquiry is greatly enlarged when it starts from an interest in disease problems as well as in environmental planning. Many examples could be cited to support the conclusion that medical interest is essential in identification and investigation of environmental influences on health, if not always in the measures needed to achieve control. It was a doctor's experience of cholera that led to investigation of the water supply; observations on the malformed resulted in recognition of the teratogenic effects of rubella and thalidomide; and a surgeon's awareness of the different disease patterns in Africans and Europeans drew attention to the significance of refinement of food to intestinal disease.

Under the reorganized National Health Service the medical role in environmental medicine is at least in danger of being weakened. Some of those working in this field will be only too pleased to be free of the medical yoke, and with medical responsibility focused on services provided under the NHS, educators are quite likely to respond by concluding that the environment has no place in medical education. Even if environmental problems are assigned to a special class of doctors, it will be difficult for such a class to emerge if the subject finds no place in undergraduate training.

I suggest that at least three steps are necessary: strengthening of the medical role in environmental medicine, with appropriate developments in training; a more co-ordinated approach to the different hazards of the environment (occupational, domestic, iatrogenic, etc.) both centrally and locally; and a considered attack on the risks associated with medical investigation and treatment.

BEHAVIOUR

The behavioural change most significant for health in the past was the limitation of family size which led to restriction of numbers. This influence is critical in developing countries today, and is still important in many developed countries whose populations have not yet achieved a rate of growth consistent with the needs of health and welfare. Nevertheless in the advanced countries it is on modification of personal habits such as smoking and sedentary living that health primarily depends.

This brings us to one of the most sensitive areas of discussion related to the health field. Many people who can accept the need for public intervention in food policies, control of environment, and provision of medical care, are deeply suspicious of attempts to modify personal behaviour. Our habits commonly begin as pleasures of which we have no need and end as necessities in which we have no pleasure. Nevertheless we tend to resent the suggestion that anyone should try to change them, even on the disarming grounds that they do so for our own good.

Two objections are often raised to the proposal that behaviour should be modified by public action: that this would be an unreasonable intrusion on the rights of the individual; and that any such attempt would be certain to fail. These objections will be examined more closely, with special reference to smoking which epitomizes the problem and the difficulties.

On the first point, it is said that the individual must be free to choose whether he wishes to smoke. But he is not free; with a drug of addiction the option is open only at the beginning, so that the critical decision to smoke is taken, not by consenting adults but by children below the age of consent. The question confronting society is not therefore whether smoking by addicts should be prohibited; it is whether it is acceptable to induce children to become addicts at an age when they neither know nor much care about the associated risks.

The same logic should be applied to other aspects of personal behaviour which are known to be important to health. It is not suggested that we should be required to exercise, to limit consumption of alcohol, sugar, and dairy products, and to avoid self-prescribed drugs and some of the physician-prescribed variety, beneficial as all these measures would undoubtedly be for our health. But it is not inconsistent with respect for personal freedom to attempt to create an environment which encourages people to do what is good for them and to avoid what is bad. It seems particularly reprehensible to do the reverse, to seek ways to induce children to damage their health by smoking for no other purpose than to sustain revenue and profits.

The conclusion that personal habits cannot be modified by acceptable public action is I think mistaken, and arises largely from the application of too short a time-scale. The physician says, 'I have not so far succeeded in persuading many, perhaps any, of my patients to give up tobacco', and he concludes that smoking habits are unchanged. Nevertheless they are visibly changing. As a lifelong non-smoker, or almost, having given up at the age of 6, for most of my life I have been a member of a depressed class. Not to smoke was often regarded as antisocial, and refusal of a cigarette at an awkward first meeting was considered equivalent to unwillingness to shake hands. I now find myself frequently in company where it would be as difficult to smoke as it was formerly not to, and where most of those present would be about as reluctant to light up in public as they would be to spit. It is not a valid objection that a change in smoking habits has so far been observed mainly in doctors, for refinements of behaviour usually begin with a sensitive or well-informed minority and spread gradually to others, an observation made by Frazer in the opening pages of *The Golden Bough*.

Moreover there is evidence that the general population is also affected. Not so long ago it was difficult to find a non-smoking compartment in a train and it was thought unreasonable to object to smoking in one. (How often one heard: 'You don't mind, do you dear?') Today half the accommodation of main-line trains in Britain is reserved for non-smokers and I have the impression that they are the most crowded compartments. About half the adult population are non-smokers, but more than half are already aware that it is unpleasant to sit in the presence of smokers.

The conclusion that behaviour changes, albeit over a longer time-scale than we might like, is well illustrated by experience of contraception. Before 1800 there was no convincing evidence that human beings would ever restrict their reproduction on a significant scale, yet by the end of the century birth-rates were falling throughout the western world. That change also began among well-informed people, but extended gradually to all sections of the population. With this evidence of modification of one of the most intimate features of behaviour there is no reason to doubt that in time other practices which are critical to health will also change.

However much thought needs to be given to the means by which such changes can be brought about. The usual approach through advertisements, posters, and public exhortations seems much too superficial, and takes little account of the subtle influences which are shaping behaviour. It is questionable whether advertisements ever led anyone to become a smoker or an alcoholic, their main influence being on the amount smoked or on the selection of a particular fag or tipple. Indeed the effect of professional advertising is probably trivial in relation to that of the variety provided gratuitously by press and television. Even the most responsible newspapers have no hesitation in exhibiting some of the most admired figures of our time with cigarettes in their hands or mouths. On 11 April 1976, the *Sunday Times* devoted nearly half a page to a photograph of Glenda Jackson as 'The Abbess', which seemed to symbolize divine as well as social sanction for the lighted cigarette suspended limply from the corner of her mouth. With unsolicited support of this kind it would not be surprising if the tobacco companies regarded their vigorous defence of paid advertising as no more than a minor skirmish designed to divert attention from the significance of the main event.

Yet if a distinguished actress cannot be persuaded to give up smoking for her own good, she might accept that she should not prejudice the health of her admirers, who include young children, by displaying her addiction in public. The same appeal might be addressed to doctors on behalf of their patients and to parents on behalf of their children. Clearly there is no general answer to the diverse problems associated with modification of behaviour except perhaps that they should be considered individually and with imagination as well as tact. Broadly what is needed is a change in way of life rather than a commentary on it, which is all that is achieved by some of the traditional methods of health education.

Finally, in health education it is necessary to reconcile three potentially conflicting aims: preservation of people's confidence in their own health; recognition of personal responsibility for maintaining health; and awareness of symptoms that require medical attention.

The first aim is the least well recognized but is arguably the most important. The individual's belief in his health is precious, but is easily shaken. With a little injudicious prompting a cheerful extrovert can be transformed into a melancholy hypochondriac, and a whole community can become preoccupied with disease when undue emphasis is placed on its precursors. This trend is already evident in the United States and Canada, where television exploits the obsession with health to promote commodities of dubious value, and every newspaper carries articles which contribute to the morbid fascination of disease. Such articles have varied origins: human interest stories ('how bravely so-and-so has borne with her disabilities'); requests for financial support for research ('help cure cancer, multiple sclerosis, rheumatism, etc.'); and appeals to the apparently well to discover disease early, promoted by screening enthusiasts. These activities are well intended, but their benefits will be bought dearly if they lead to a general loss of confidence in personal health.

Some risks are also associated with the otherwise unexceptionable efforts to persuade people to look after their health by modifying personal behaviour. There are no obvious disadvantages in presenting smoking as a practice analogous rather than homologous to spitting, equally unpleasant but much more lethal; or in suggesting that physical exercise and control of weight advance the quality as well as the duration of life. But when along with such advice people are encouraged to monitor their weight, pulse and blood pressure, we are in some danger of crossing the delicate line which divides a quiet confidence in health from a morbid preoccupation with its loss.

It is even more difficult to dissociate anxiety from awareness of symptoms that require medical attention. On the whole it would be better if the public realized that most acute respiratory and intestinal disorders have no serious significance and do not require investigation and treatment; the same cannot be said about lumps in the breast, chest pain related to effort, and unexplained bleeding from the lower orifices. Perhaps the most difficult task for health education is to reconcile awareness of the need for investigation of such symptoms with preservation of people's confidence in their own health.

Some of the same problems arise in relation to screening for early evidence of disease. Let us consider as an example the proposal, widely supported, to introduce mass screening for hypertension. The evidence appears to show that treatment of hypertension prevents, or more probably postpones, some deaths from stroke and heart failure but not from coronary artery disease. However, before deciding that this observation should lead to screening of the general population for raised blood pressure we should recognize the difficulties involved. When people are identified as hypertensives by mass screening, because of the unreliability of the measurement some are incorrectly diagnosed; some who are correctly diagnosed do not follow the prescribed treatment; in some who follow the treatment, control of pressure is not achieved; and some are treated unnecessarily, because there are people whose high pressure appears to be compatible with a life of normal duration and quality. But perhaps the most serious consideration is that the quality of life is gravely prejudiced for many people when they are told that they have a life-threatening condition of which they were previously unaware. (An investigation in industry has shown that absentee rates are nearly doubled among workers when they are informed that they have raised blood pressure.)[4] Hence for those who get some benefit from screening, a much larger number pay a considerable price in anxiety and harmful side-effects of drugs.

THE EVIDENCE REQUIRED FOR PUBLIC ACTION

It is sometimes suggested that action cannot be taken to modify influences which may promote or damage health until evidence of their effects is complete. For this reason some would say that it would be unacceptable to change national food policies, to prohibit certain kinds of television advertising, to control suspected hazards in industry, to restrict the use of potentially dangerous drugs or to attempt to modify

4. Haynes, R. B., Sackett, D. L., Taylor, D. W., Gibson, E. S. and Johnson, A. L., 'Absenteeism from work after the detection and labelling of hypertensives', *The New England Journal of Medicine*, 299, No. 14 (1978), p. 741.

behaviour, except possibly in the case of cigarette smoking where the grounds are considered to be sufficient.

It is fortunate that this requirement was not always imposed in the past. When Snow protected a London population from cholera in the mid nineteenth century by removing the handle of the Broad Street pump, the evidence of the relation between the disease and the water supply was anything but complete; indeed neither micro-organisms nor tests of significance had been discovered. If thalidomide had not been withdrawn on the basis of an observed association between the drug and limb deformities and when knowledge of teratogenesis was very deficient (as it still is), many thousands of children would have been born with malformations. If the argument that an association does not prove causation and only experimental evidence is conclusive had been accepted, quite a number of people who found the relation between cigarette smoking and lung cancer sufficiently convincing would have died of the disease before beagles had been taught to smoke. And during the last war, if the limited foods then available had not been distributed judiciously by rationing, subsidies and supplements, the health of the population would have been much less satisfactory than in fact it was. Yet it was not then, nor is it now, possible to specify with any precision the nature and mode of operation of the nutritional influences which were important.

Other examples could be cited in support of the view that action is often needed to protect and promote health in circumstances where the evidence is less than complete. Moreover, in many cases it is questionable whether within the foreseeable future the evidence will be complete. To assess precisely the respective roles of diet, exercise and smoking in the causation of coronary artery disease, a massive human experiment would be needed, with division of a population into multiple experimental and control groups. Such an investigation would present formidable ethical, technical and administrative difficulties. Does this mean that no action can be taken in this and similar cases because the grounds, however suggestive, are not conclusive?

In the light of such difficulties I believe it will often be desirable to act on the basis of high, or even moderate, probabilities, on what has been called 'a burden of prudence' rather than 'a burden of proof'. When applying this principle, however, we should distinguish between the levels of proof needed for private and for public actions. Parents can act to protect their own or their children's health on evidence which would not be considered sufficient to justify public action. For example, they might think it right to encourage their children not to smoke, to avoid white bread and to limit their consumption of foods and drinks containing sugar, at a time when none of these practices is publicly prohibited. The level of proof needed for public action is a different question and has no single answer. Nevertheless, it should be recognized that conclusive evidence of harm or benefit to health is often an unrealistic requirement.

Clinical Services

The conclusion that medical intervention has made, and can be expected to make a relatively small contribution to prevention of sickness and death could not fail to have large implications for personal health services. They have evolved on quite different assumptions; treatment by surgery and drugs is widely regarded as the basis of health and the essence of medical care, and nearly half of the total expenditure in Britain (46.0 per cent in 1970/1) is on acute hospitals. These hospitals do not care for most sick people, of whom the large majority are in their own homes under general practitioners or in psychiatric, geriatric, or other institutions.

There are many issues which arise from reappraisal of the determinants of health but I shall limit my comment to four which are particularly important: the tasks of clinical medicine; the relation between technology and care; the problem of ensuring the quality of care; and the relation between medically qualified and other health workers.

THE TASKS OF CLINICAL MEDICINE

It is no criticism of clinical medicine to say that it has less effect than non-personal and behavioural influences on indices such as death-rates and expectation of life. But does it follow that these yardsticks are inappropriate to the work of the clinician? This view has been stated as follows: 'Today's often repeated cliché that what the physician does has relatively little influence on health is more correctly stated that what the physician does has relatively little influence on those indicators of health that are largely irrelevant to what he does.' And 'the great difference between measuring quality in the public health system, in which it can be reckoned by changes in disease pattern, and in the personal – encounter – physician system, in which it is a matter of the appropriateness of a human act: so-called "outcome" results are obtainable in the former, but as a practical matter are seldom helpful in the latter'.[1]

This conclusion is drawn largely from recognition of two difficulties, one of assessing the effectiveness of the work of the personal doctor, and the other of separating it from other responsibilities for patient care, sometimes referred to as the samaritan or pastoral role.

Recognizing these difficulties, I nevertheless think it is important to examine the different components of clinical service before concluding that indices of effectiveness are irrelevant to them. Not indeed with the idea that all items of service can be assessed accurately, or that they can be dissociated from one another in the day-to-day delivery of care. But sooner rather than later, rising costs will make it necessary to introduce cost/benefit assessment, and for this it will be essential to classify clinical services according to the nature of the tasks involved. Without this preliminary classification it would be very difficult to evaluate the work done in an acute medical ward (which may range from reassurance to care of an unconscious patient in the last hours of life), and impossible to compare the value of the very different services rendered to, say, a surgical patient, a pregnant woman and a subnormal child.

There is another reason for attempting to clarify the tasks of clinical medicine. Remarkably, considering that one of the reasons given for not assessing outcome is the importance of the samaritan role, it is the samaritan role itself which is often prejudiced by lack of evidence of effectiveness. For when clinical procedures are not evaluated scientifically, they are evaluated intuitively; each practitioner makes up his own mind about the usefulness of, say, radical mastectomy, tonsillectomy, cervical cytology and prolonged rest after myocardial infarction. The benefits of intervention and the associated technology are frequently overestimated, and this may result in the neglect of patients after the acute phase of illness, or of those (such as the subnormal) who provide no scope for active measures.

A satisfactory classification of the tasks is not yet in sight, and I can say for the one that follows only that it is the best I have been able to devise and has seemed acceptable to clinical colleagues with whom I have discussed it. I suggest that the services can be considered under five headings: reassurance; treatment of an acute emergency; cure; care; and comfort.

1. McDermott, W., 'Evaluating the physician and his technology', in *Daedalus*, 106 (1977), No. 1, p. 155.

REASSURANCE

If we exclude those who take 'cures' with no wish to be cured, one of the most welcome clinical services is reassurance that the patient's fears are ill founded. Most people who believe themselves to be ill have in common their need for reassurance and sympathy, a point illustrated charmingly in Proust's novel by his account of his aunt Léonie. She was a hypochondriac who had restricted her life, first to her house, later to her bedroom, and finally to her bed, where she devoted herself entirely to her two interests, her health and her religion. She placed her medicines and a statue of Our Lady on a table which served a dual function as pharmacy and high altar, and she dismissed from her company two classes of people: those who said there was nothing wrong with her (they were unsympathetic) and those who took her health at her own morbid evaluation (they failed to reassure her). But to provide reassurance in an acceptable form is not always easy; Aunt Léonie did not like to be told that she would live to be a hundred, 'for she preferred to have no definite limit fixed to the number of her days'.

In the present context it should be noted that all medical reassurance is not equally well founded. After pathological examination of a lump from the breast, a patient can be told confidently that there is no evidence of malignancy; the same confidence may not be justified when it is said that digestive symptoms have no serious significance.

TREATMENT OF AN ACUTE EMERGENCY

Under this heading, I refer to emergencies which are usually life-threatening: for example, a serious accident; obstructed labour; stroke; coronary thrombosis. Although many of the conditions which lead to such emergencies also present a medium or long-term threat to the duration or quality of life (discussed below under 'cure'), the handling of the acute condition is of such importance that it deserves to be evaluated in its own right. For the patient and close relatives other considerations are secondary until the immediate crisis has passed.

This is an aspect of clinical service in which the test of benefit or outcome seems entirely appropriate. It is surely important to be aware that medical intervention is very successful in many, probably most, acute emergencies; that it has limited success in others (for example, it has been estimated that at best it can influence the survival of about half the patients admitted to hospital with coronary thrombosis who would otherwise die from the acute attack); and that it may have little or no effect on the immediately outcome, as in the case of stroke.

CURE

I refer here to the treatment of all conditions which threaten the duration or quality of life. Acute emergencies are excluded, but not the residual diseases or disabilities which remain after they have passed.

Defined in this way the diseases in which cure is an appropriate aim vary greatly in type and severity. They may affect the quality of life or its duration or both. They include, to illustrate their range, the common cold and the psychoses, as examples of the first; and typhoid and neoplastic disease as examples of the second.

It is not a criticism of medical research and practice that many conditions cannot be cured in the sense that the patient's health is completely restored. Nor do I overlook the problems of estimating the outcome of treatment. But the difficulty of achieving or assessing benefit should not blind us to its central place among clinical services. The pianist who has lost the use of a hand as a result of a stroke, and the cellist crippled by multiple sclerosis are in no doubt about the assistance they would most welcome, the restoration of both the duration and the quality of life. (The cruel nature of the disability in such cases sometimes tempts one to think, in very unscientific terms, that it is the site of injury rather than its extent which demonstrates the malignancy of fate: Degas blind, Beethoven deaf and Johnson dumb.)

This is perhaps a suitable point at which to refer to the normal expectation of life which medicine should aim to restore. Early in this century Osler's reference to 'chloroform at sixty' in a famous speech was an indication of the age at which life was thought to be more or less completed (very different from Sarah Bernhardt's reply when, aged eight-four, she was asked at what age women lose interest in men: 'You must ask an old woman.') Today many people, including some experienced clinicians, speak in much the same way of age seventy, influenced no doubt by the fact that this is about the expectation of life at birth for the sexes combined in developed countries. However, life expectation is lowered by many potentially preventable deaths in early and middle life, and for those who avoid such accidents, it is considerably longer. On the basis of present estimates for developed countries, if people who are congenitally handicapped are excluded, the genetically determined expectation of life at birth appears to be a little under eighty for males and a little over for females.

CARE AND COMFORT

Under the samaritan or pastoral role I include all services, other than
investigation and treatment, which are needed during acute illness,
during convalescence, and for prolonged periods, in some cases for the
rest of their lives, by chronically ill or handicapped people. Within this
framework it is useful to distinguish between care and comfort. Under
care I am thinking of a wide range of services, from washing, dressing,
feeding and lifting of bedridden patients to the education and training
of handicapped people. These services are provided largely by health
workers other than doctors, most of whom require professional or
semi-professional training. Under comfort, I refer to personal sympathy
and support, as distinguished from specific services. This is provided
largely by the patient's relatives and close friends; nevertheless by virtue
of his medical role the doctor has a unique responsibility in relation
to it.

It should be noted that the preceding discussion has been written with
reference to services to the patient (cure, care, comfort, etc.) and not
to the means (diagnosis, investigation, etc.) that are needed to perform
the service. Although I should not wish to defend the details of the
classification too vigorously, I believe that medicine requires an analysis
of this kind. It is necessary as a prerequisite to cost/benefit assessment
to identify those tasks in which appraisal of benefit is appropriate and
to ensure that the importance of the samaritan role is not overlooked
because of misconceptions about achievements under other headings.

TECHNOLOGY AND CARE

Since the eighteenth century medical activities have been divided
broadly into favoured and depressed areas corresponding respectively
to patients for whom it was thought something could be done and
others, the large majority, for whom little could be done. This distinction had its origin in the admission policies of voluntary hospitals.
Although their work was not originally restricted, from the eighteenth
century it became increasingly concerned with short-term care. This
made it necessary for public authorities to accept responsibility for other
classes of patients.

In Britain the decision to make admission to an institution a condition
of public assistance (in 1834) brought the large number of destitute sick

under the Poor Law. They were accommodated in workhouses, supplemented later by infirmaries built as hospitals. But the infirmaries,following the example of the voluntary hospitals, restricted their admissions, and the medical care of the indigent was left to the mixed workhouse, the only institution unable to reject it. This grouping of a large heterogeneous class of patients who had in common only their destitution was the origin of the chronic hospital.

From the nineteenth century the mentally ill, also excluded from the voluntary hospitals, were admitted to county asylums. This separated them from the Poor Law, and led to a division of responsibility between mental and chronic hospitals. Finally the establishment of acute psychiatric units in general hospitals further exaggerated the isolation of the mental hospital. The history of institutions for the mentally subnormal is in some respects parallel. This is the background of the most significant feature of hospitals, the separation of mental, chronic (now geriatric), and mental subnormality hospitals from general hospitals.

The distinction between hospitals had its parallel in a division of medical practice. The founding of voluntary hospitals from the eighteenth century, and of public hospitals from the nineteenth had two very significant effects: it changed what had been wholly a domiciliary service into one in which hospital work became increasingly important; and it replaced the long-standing divisions between physician, surgeon, and apothecary by another between general practitioner and consultant. Originally this distinction had little justification in their training and competence, and was determined mainly by their relationship to the hospital. In the words of the *British Medical Journal*, a consultant was 'a practitioner among the sick who could charge higher fees because he had a hospital appointment'. Even today, the consultant is distinguished from the general practitioner less by the subtlety of his treatment than by the strength of conviction with which he executes it.

The division of medical work into favoured and depressed areas which has existed since the eighteenth century is in danger of being extended by the growth of technology. Professional interest is increasingly absorbed by methods of investigation and treatment whose complexities seem to challenge the attention of the best minds and whose rewards are assumed to justify it. The acute hospital is likely to become still more selective in its admission policies, and the teaching centre with its concentration of resources and abilities, will be the most exclusive of all. Doctors, nurses, and other health workers would then be trained in an environment which reveals a very limited part of the health task, an environment where prestige, rewards, and professional interest all seem to point in the same direction. After qualification, understandably, they will seek to continue in the activities which were the focus of their training, and only with the greatest reluctance will they consent to enter the massive neglected areas of health care. The large number of patients, particularly among the congenitally handicapped, the mentally ill and the aged sick, whose disabilities are not thought to provide scope for technology, will be pushed further into the background, and the division of health services into two worlds will be even sharper than it is today.

Many people who regret this trend, and particularly the low standards of care for the majority of patients to which it leads, nevertheless think it is justified by the achievements of acute hospitals. They suggest that if a choice must be made it is better to treat appendicitis in a young adult before incontinence in an elderly person. However, such examples are entirely misleading. In the first place, mean age of admissions has risen in the past thirty years, and a comparison between patients in acute and other hospitals is now mainly between the old and the old, rather than between the young and the old. Secondly, a successful operation which restores the patient to health is not typical of the work of acute hospitals, much of which is palliative or unproved. Thirdly, in what is unsatisfactorily referred to as the chronic sector there is scope for services which are as critical to health as any on the acute side. Consider, for example, the need to admit to an institution a hyperactive mentally retarded child who is destroying the health as well as the happiness of the family. Such children are to be found in every large town; yet their care is not regarded as urgent and is rarely given the priority it merits on health grounds.

A recent reaction to the disparity of standards is the proposal that it should be adjusted by a transfer of resources from acute to chronic care. However, the matter is more complex than this approach suggests. Acute services are not all of a kind: some are among the most effective measures that medicine can offer and any reduction of support would be deplorable; others have never been evaluated; still others are known to be ineffective and undoubtedly waste resources. What is needed is a more accurate mapping of the effectiveness and efficiency of services, an approach more readily applied to new developments than to existing procedures.

Moreover, the needs of so-called chronic patients will not be met simply by an increase in expenditure, and indeed the terms acute and chronic are themselves misleading. Patients do not fall sharply into two classes according to their need for technology or care; those in general hospitals need personal care, and many in mental, geriatric and subnormality hospitals would benefit from investigation and treatment. Furthermore, with a population of hospital patients composed mainly of the elderly, as is the case today, the different phases of care (acute, rehabilitative, prolonged) are required by the same people at different stages of their lives and sometimes at different stages of the same episode of illness.

What is needed is a re-thinking of the whole framework of services (hospitals, medical practice, and community health and social services) in the light of the conclusion that the task confronting the personal health services is the complete care of patients, using that term in the widest sense to include active rehabilitation, prolonged and terminal care, as well as investigation and treatment of acute illness. In broad terms what is required is a framework which meets, and where necessary reconciles, the diverse need of technology and care.[2] This aim is unlikely to be achieved under a fragmented hospital system which isolates the majority of patients (mental, geriatric, and subnormal) from the resources of the general hospital, or in a system of medical practice in which the hospital work of the general practitioner is separated (in community hospitals) from the work of the consultant.

QUALITY OF CARE

Since there is some confusion over terminology I should make it clear that I am using the term quality of care comprehensively to include (a) standard of care (how well we do what we do), (b) effectiveness of care (whether what we do is worth doing), and (c) efficiency of care (whether what we do makes better use of resources than the available alternatives).

Standard of care, as I conceive it, is concerned with appraisal of existing practices: by an individual, a profession, or an institution such as a hospital or health centre. It is not concerned with the usefulness of the services rendered nor with the cost/benefit issues which arise in relation to efficiency. Appraisal of standards may require assessment of the adequacy of facilities: buildings, equipment, etc., sometimes referred to as structure; or of the operation of services, sometimes described as

2. I have described the kind of hospital that would meet these requirements (a balanced hospital community) in *Medicine in Modern Society* (London: George Allen and Unwin Ltd, 1965).

process. Examination of standards has been relatively uncommon in Britain, largely because of conservative traditions, particularly the professional independence of the individual practitioner and consultant; it is more frequent in the United States where doctors are often willing to examine, and to have others examine critically, the standard of their work. Improvement in standards depends largely on the education and graduate training of doctors, and on the decision of professional organizations such as the Royal Colleges to take the subject very seriously.

I am using the terms effectiveness and efficiency essentially in the sense that Cochrane employed them, in reference not only to preventive and therapeutic measures such as vaccines, drugs, and surgery, but also to various features of the organization of care such as duration of stay in hospital and evaluation of home and hospital care. He emphasized particularly the use of randomized controlled trials in such assessments. All that need be added here is that the organization of the necessary investigations may be extremely complex, since they may require large-scale research involving several centres and continuing over a prolonged period. They may also be restricted by ethical considerations. One need think only of the problems arising currently in evaluation of screening for breast cancer to appreciate the difficulties. To those associated with assessment of effectiveness, appraisal of efficiency adds the further complication of estimation of *relative* benefits and costs of different procedures. However, I think it can be said without complacency that in examination of effectiveness at least, work in Britain compares not unfavourably with that in other countries. If we are cautious about evaluating how well we do what we do, we are at least fairly ready to consider whether it is worth doing.

However, the main point to be made about the quality of care in the present context is a different one. We have overestimated the effectiveness of many procedures and services in current use, and indeed most have been adopted without adequate evaluation. It is important now, and with rising costs it will be imperative in future, to adopt a far more critical approach to appraisal of the various facets of quality: standard, effectiveness, and efficiency. Medicine must be prepared to face the tests which are inescapable in private enterprise and which it is almost unique among public activities in having evaded hitherto: Is our work well done? Is it worth doing? and Does it pay its way?

No one familiar with the problems associated with these assessments in medicine can be in any doubt about the difficulties, particularly in the case of procedures and services already in use. Once a procedure has come into general use it may be difficult, perhaps impossible to withdraw it after facilities have been provided, staff trained, and public expectations roused. However, there is a point in time when a new measure is sufficiently promising to justify its introduction on a limited scale, and when it is not yet so widely used that there are ethical and other objections to investigation of its effectiveness. If this opportunity is missed it cannot easily be recreated, and it is for this reason that it is now difficult or impossible to assess the value of many procedures and services which have never been validated. There are, however, a few examples in recent years where a critical appraisal was made at the appropriate time, in clinical trials of vaccines and, more recently, in evaluation of screening procedures. There is little doubt that if this approach had not been adopted we should by now be committed to a breast cancer screening service of large cost, limited benefit, and unknown risks.

In the case of standards of care, given professional understanding and co-operation there should be no insuperable difficulty in improving existing procedures. But in consideration of effectiveness and efficiency attention should be focused particularly on new developments. Methods of investigation and treatment are likely to become more complex, costly, and, in some cases, hazardous than in the past. It should be the aim of policy to achieve control of such developments, and to ensure that no new procedure comes into general use until its benefits and costs have been estimated and its risks are known. These requirements apply to services in general; but they should be particularly stringent in the case of protective services such as screening. When people who believe themselves to be well are invited to submit to examination they should be assured not only that they may benefit but also that they are not being exposed to unknown risks.

MEDICAL AND OTHER HEALTH WORKERS

In providing medical care the doctor has long relied on the co-operation of other workers, for example, in earlier centuries the apothecary who made up his prescriptions, and more recently the nurse who attends to his patients for much of the time when he is otherwise engaged. But in the twentieth century, and particularly the last few decades, there has been a large increase in the number of professionals and para-professionals who contribute to health care, and their relation to the doctor and to one another has become a major issue. Trade unionism, women's rights, professional prestige, and no doubt several other less readily specified influences have been at work, and the idea that the doctor is the natural leader of the health team, the person directly responsible to the patient for the effectiveness of his care in all circumstances, is no longer unchallenged.

This is not a new phenomenon; but it has become more significant. In Britain it has led to segregation from the medical services of social workers concerned with the sick, first in a separate department of local government and, since the reorganization of the NHS, under a separate authority. The environmental health officers of local authorities are no longer responsible to the medically qualified specialist who now serves as a consultant. And in the reorganized service, the objections of other health workers to medical dominance have been met by the concept of administration by consensus, a system of management designed to ensure that no one is managed. But in their relation to doctors the most important other professionals are undoubtedly nurses. In Britain they have so far accepted their traditional role with few complaints; however, in the United States nurses have asserted their independence by going their own way, and their training and role are now determined with little reference to medical tradition or opinion. In that country it might be said of doctors and nurses, as of two potential rivals, that they get on excellently because (in concepts and planning) they never meet.

The difficulties of professional relationships have existed for some time in the health field; but reaction to the doctor's position has been muted to some extent by the belief that his role is critical for the health of patients. Once it is realized that the determinants of health are largely outside the system, and that the main contribution required from personal health services is the care of the sick (using the term in its fullest sense), questions concerning medical dominance are likely to become even more insistent. Are the traditional roles of doctors and nurses appropriate in primary care, where the nurse appears to be capable of giving a service which in some countries the physician seems unable or unwilling to provide? Are responsibilities allocated sensibly in the acute ward, where it is the nurse rather than the doctor who is likely to be present at the time of serious emergencies? If the doctor is in charge in acute illness, does it follow that he should also be responsible in mental and chronic disease, where the patient's needs may be of an entirely different character? Is there a definable area of administration in which a medical qualification is essential, or should administrators, particularly senior ones, be selected as in other fields on the basis of personal gifts and experience which override technical qualifications?

These questions are not new; but they are given considerable urgency by a different reading of the determinants of health. If we accept that someone needs to be in charge of patient care and of administration of health services, it can no longer be assumed to be an automatic right of the doctor in all circumstances.

Medical Education

In this chapter I shall suggest that the aims of medical education should be broader than they are at present; that it should be concerned with all the influences on health, non-personal as well as personal, and that in the field of patient care attention should be extended to all types of patients and all phases of illness.

A proposal of this kind is certain to provoke what many will regard as an insuperable objection. It will be said that patients come to doctors for assistance when they are unwell, and that the essential medical function is to meet this need; it is regrettable if this leads to some loss of interest in other influences on health and in the less active phases of care, but neither is exclusively a medical responsibility and this is a price which must be paid for concentration on the most important task: the diagnosis and treatment of disease in individual patients.

This is the logic which explains and is thought to justify the somewhat restricted aims of medical education. In challenging the conclusions two things must be shown: first, that 'other influences' are critical for health and require medical participation; and second, that when the diagnosis and treatment of disease is considered to be the only medical functions, many patients' needs are neglected.

THE CASE FOR WIDER AIMS

OTHER INFLUENCES ON HEALTH

Their importance has been discussed at some length and the conclusions can be summarized by saying that health was transformed from the eighteenth century because of improved nutrition, better hygiene, and contraception, and without a significant contribution from immunization and treatment before the twentieth century; and although the point is purely theoretical, it is unlikely that medical intervention would have been effective if the other advances had not occurred.

In assessing the medical contribution which is needed a distinction must be made between environmental influences, which are essentially non-personal, and behavioural influences which are largely of a personal character.

Environmental influences. The grounds for retaining and extending the medical contribution to environmental medicine were outlined in Chapter 9. They are essentially the importance of the field, and the fact that although doctors often have little to contribute to the control of recognized hazards, identification of additional ones frequently results from observation of patients. In the case of hazards associated with investigation and treatment of disease, both recognition and control are almost inconceivable without medical participation.

The contribution of doctors to environmental medicine is of two kinds which have implications for medical education and postgraduate training. First, doctors in practice should be equipped to advise their patients about risks which may arise in relation to work, travel, domestic circumstances, and, occasionally, recreation. Second, medical specialists are needed who can contribute to investigation and control of hazards in all the main areas in which they arise: local, national, occupational, and medical. While some specialists may restrict their work to a particular area such as occupational health, it seems desirable that they should be trained basically in all aspects of environmental medicine, and that they should be identified professionally with other specialists who work in the same field.

Behavioural influences. In developed countries these are now the predominant determinants of health. In the past, modification of personal behaviour for health purposes was by the conventional forms of health education, a task assigned largely to non-medical people and one in which doctors on the whole took little interest. These arrangements had serious disadvantages: they separated assessment of unhealthy behaviour (undertaken mainly by research workers) from public communication (in the hands of professional educators); they placed the emphasis on an approach through posters, advertising, and public exhortation rather than through more subtle and complex modifications of ways of life; and they seemed to remove responsibility for health education from doctors in practice, who are often in the best position to influence the behaviour of their patients. More vigorous medical participation is needed, and is unlikely to be achieved if the significance of personal behaviour, and the role of the doctor in relation to it, are not given sufficient attention in medical education.

AN EXTENDED CONCEPT OF MEDICAL CARE

In some respects more serious than the effect on other influences is the restricted concept of personal care which results from identification of diagnosis and treatment as the only medical function. In hospital and consultant services it has led to the relative neglect of the majority of patients (the mentally ill, the subnormal, and the aged sick) who are not thought to provide scope for the investigative and therapeutic procedures which are the main concern of the acute hospitals. In Britain the deficiency is now well recognized; but the solution advocated is often a simple diversion of resources to the neglected areas, rather than a new approach to the whole relation between short-, intermediate-, and long-term care. It was suggested above (Chapter 10) that this is unlikely to be achieved by a hospital system which places different classes of patients in separate institutions.

Moreover the deficiencies of care are not restricted to those who are severley handicapped by mental illness, subnormality, or extreme age. Patients who are well cared for so long as they are under active investigation and treatment are often neglected during the later stages of their illness, particularly if these are protracted. Since the eighteenth century general hospitals have sought to avoid admission of those who are likely to outstay their welcome, and if after completion of active measures patients have not recovered sufficiently to return home, they are, if possible, discharged to other institutions. In some countries the deficiencies go even further, and a patient with an incurable illness is no longer of much interest to the doctor who made the diagnosis. The lesson has not yet been learned everywhere that diagnosis of disease is of little value if it does not lead to effective treatment or care, and in general (there are some necessary exceptions) care at different stages of an illness should not be divided between doctors and between institutions.

It will of course be said, and rightly, that in Britain these criticisms are more applicable to hospitals than to general practice, that many general practitioners provide prolonged care, including terminal care of patients in their own homes. At its best this service works reasonably well for domiciliary care; but it sometimes not at its best, it is not available in hospitals, and in some countries it is not available at all. The general criticism remains valid; in medicine in the late twentieth century exaggeration of the contribution of investigation and treatment of disease leads to serious neglect of the substantial and continuing needs of many patients.

If interest is to be extended to non-personal influences on health and to all phases of care, changes will be needed in medical education. The conclusions must be considered in relation to selection of students, the medical curriculum, and the image of medicine projected at the teaching centre.

SELECTION OF STUDENTS

From time to time the question is asked whether the right people come into medicine; and although it is usually unanswered, or inconclusively answered, perhaps it should be considered again whenever changes are proposed in the role and education of the doctor. My own experience of admission procedures, happily quite brief, was sufficient to convince me that Shaw's comment early in the century remains valid: 'Unless a man is led to medicine or surgery through a very exceptional technical aptitude, or because doctoring is a family tradition, or because he regards it unintelligently as a lucrative and gentlemanly profession, his motives in choosing the career of a healer are clearly generous.'[1] Perhaps today the exceptions should also include some who are influenced by examination success in the so-called basic sciences (physics, chemistry, biology, and mathematics) which many school and university teachers consider to be the best evidence of suitability for a career in medicine. (In the present context it is significant that medical schools often place more emphasis on physical than on biological science.) However, there is no reason to doubt that most entrants to medical schools are strongly, and on the whole, generously motivated.

There is also no reason to question their intellectual abilities. Except in those unfortunate countries which have to accept all qualified students into the first year, medical schools everywhere have a high ratio of applicants to admission places. Since all university applications are

1. Preface to *The Doctor's Dilemma*.

assessed in much the same way, in Britain largely on results of 'O'-
and 'A'-level examinations, students admitted to medical schools are
probably as least as able as those entering other professions. Medicine
cannot ask for more.

However, students undoubtedly come into medicine with some very
definite ideas about the career on which they are embarking and the
training appropriate for it. Their ideas reflect the predominant notions
in society about the work of the doctor: that he is concerned with the
diagnosis and treatment of disease in individual patients, that most
patients are cured by treatment and that it is on medical intervention
that health primarily depends. It is like a slap on the face for a student
to be told at the outset of his training that at least on the second and
third points these ideas need revision: that health is not determined
mainly by medical intervention and that the needs of patients extend
far beyond what can be achieved by investigation and active treatment.

When these concepts are widely known it is possible that they may
have some influence on the decision of students to select medicine as a
career; applicants should perhaps be drawn more frequently than at
present from the two ends of a spectrum of interest from which recruitment is largely from the middle. An identikit of the contemporary
medical student would be one who combines aptitude for physical and
biological science with concern about the care of individual patients.
But his interest in medical science is not such that he would wish to
pursue it if it led away from personal care; and his concern about personal care is not strong enough for him to devote himself to it if divorced
from investigation and active treatment. There is undoubtedly a larger
place for people who are interested in the application of medical science
through measures such as nutrition, environment, and population control, but who would not wish to undertake personal care; and for
physicians who are selected primarily for their interest and concern for
the welfare of patients, including those who are permanently handicapped. Such applicants are not easily recognized, but in the course of
time, as the public image of medicine is modified, they may select themselves.

But although medicine would undoubtedly benefit from recruitment
of some students who at present are more likely to find their way into
engineering or social service, I do not think that the difficulty of training
doctors to meet the needs of society arises because the wrong people
are chosen. The students who enter medical schools are reasonably able
and, in spite of some remarkable exceptions, generously motivated, and

their idea of the determinants of health and of the doctor's role is only a reflection of the current views of society. The failure to enlarge the concept of the medical task (and the loss of motivation, where it occurs) are usually due to subsequent training, to what they hear and see during the years in a medical school and teaching hospital. The important influences are the medical curriculum and the image of medicine projected at the teaching hospital.

THE MEDICAL CURRICULUM

Although students are probably more influenced by the practice and research of the teaching centre than by what they hear in lectures and seminars, the medical curriculum is important, not least as an indication of the subjects and methods which are considered relevant to the education of a doctor. While there is some variation from school to school, and considerable variation from country to country, there is no serious dispute about the basic concepts; medicine is thought to be concerned with intervention in disease processes, mainly by investigation and treatment of established disease, but also by immunization against infections and, to a limited extent, by early recognition of disease through screening. Since the intervention is by physical, chemical, and biological methods it is not surprising that the basic sciences are considered to be physics, chemistry, and biology; that medical education begins with study of the structure and function of the body (anatomy, physiology, and biochemistry); that it continues with examination of disease processes (pathology and microbiology); and that it ends with clinical instruction on selected patients of the types seen in a teaching hospital.

The limitations of this approach were discussed in Chapter 2. The preoccupation with disease mechanisms leads away from consideration of the underlying causes of disease whose control is the essential basis of health. More surprisingly, considering that interest is focused on the sick patient, the approach also results in failure to assess critically the effectiveness of medical intervention, and to consider adequately patients' needs which are additional to investigation and active treatment.

The following are among changes needed in medical education to enlarge the concepts of health and disease and the role of medicine arising from them.

1. At the outset it should be recognized that the most fundamental

question in medicine is why disease occurs rather than how it operates after it has occurred; that is to say, conceptually the origins of disease should take precedence over the nature of disease processes. The starting point in education should therefore be the distinction between diseases established irreversibly at fertilization and those which are not, and the instruction should be concerned with genes and chromosomes, with the prenatal environment and with the wide range of post-natal influences on health, both physical and mental. It would be desirable to consider also the disease experience of early man and of other animals in their natural habitats. Considerable attention should be given to matters which have been examined in a very preliminary way in this book: the nature of the influences which have brought about the transformation in human health, and of those which may be expected to be effective in dealing with the residual health problems of developed countries.

These are not matters to be dealt with and dismissed in a series of lectures, although no doubt there is a place for a course or courses related to them. The conclusion that human health is determined by the conditions under which disease occurs is one which should influence all stages of teaching. In the early years it should enlarge the mechanistic approach in the pre-clinical departments; in the intermediate period it should complement the teaching of the pathological sciences; and in clinical medicine it should lead to a more searching discussion of disease origins in relation to individual patients.

2. In clinical teaching discussion is focused on investigation, diagnosis, pathogenesis, clinical manifestations, and treatment of disease. Questions which usually receive insufficient attention are: Why is the patient ill? How effective is the treatment and what risks are associated with it? What advice and care are needed, by the patient or his relatives after completion of active measures?

The attention given to disease origins varies from one field of medicine to another and from consultant to consultant within the same field. In general, this subject is considered more fully by physicians than by surgeons, and, understandably, by surgeons concerned with cold surgery than by those dealing mainly with acute cases. Moreover the time devoted to the origins of disease is increasing, if slowly, and some teachers review comprehensively what is known about aetiology. Nevertheless, this subject does not have the central place in clinical teaching that its importance merits; and understandably, since the essential tasks of the doctor are considered to be diagnosis and treatment. In these circumstances it is disease mechanisms rather than disease origins which provide the basis for discussion – How does the disease operate, so that we may intervene? rather than – What are the conditions which lead to it, so that we may remove them? It is surely unnecessary to add that in emphasizing the importance of the second question one is not suggesting that the first should be neglected. But the origin of disease deserves consideration even where it is unknown, for example in relation to many problems unresolved at the present time: multiple sclerosis, diabetes, Parkinsonism, schizophrenia, varicose veins, etc., as well as such ill-defined conditions as backache and the multiple forms of rheumatism. The purpose of raising these uncomfortable issues is twofold: to make doctors in practice acutely aware of the extent and limitations of knowledge of the causes (as well as the mechanisms) of disease; and to lead future research workers to reflect on the outstanding problems on the basis of something more than the conventional mechanistic approach.

3. The question concerning the effectiveness and risks of intervention can be raised with advantage on almost every patient. Again it must be said that some teachers do consider it, and a few regard it as of outstanding importance; but in general, the value and hazards of investigation and treatment are not discussed critically, and doctors complete their education with only vague ideas about the credentials of many of the tools they are expected to apply. The basic difficulty is of course, as Cochrane has emphasized,[2] that the effectiveness of most clinical procedures has never been adequately assessed; but what is not known, as well as what is known, should be made explicit in clinical teaching. To give one example: since only a minority of practising doctors are surgeons (and they train for the specialty as graduates), and a majority have to give advice from time to time about the value of surgical procedures, consideration of outcome in library, ward rounds, and seminars is more relevant to their needs than time spent in operating theatres.

4. Probably the most serious deficiency in clinical teaching is in respect of the care needed by patients after completion of investigation and treatment, and by those, the majority of all hospital patients, who are not considered to provide scope for active measures and so are never seen in teaching hospitals. This deficiency is attributable more to the limited range of work of the teaching hospital (discussed below) than to clinical teaching. Nevertheless the emphasis on investigation and

2. Cochrane, A. L., *Effectiveness and Efficiency*, Rock Carling Monograph, 1971 (Nuffield Provincial Hospitals Trust, 1972).

acute care inevitably gives students the impression that the later needs of patients, less dramatic but no less important, are a secondary consideration which can often be left to someone else. It leads to the remarkable notions that the diagnosis of a disease which cannot be treated is an end in itself, and that treatment of acute illness in an elderly person can be divorced from rehabilitative measures and prolonged care.

Any comment on the deficiencies of medical education is open to the criticism that it is not equally true of all subjects and of all teachers. And of course, it is not; there are some who consider carefully the origins of disease and the effectiveness and hazards of treatment, although they must find it almost impossible to deal convincingly with the later phases of care or with permanently handicapped people within the confines of a teaching hospital. In view of this difficulty most medical schools have introduced instruction in general practice, which extends students' experience to domiciliary care and, to a limited extent, to the later stages of illness. Nevertheless the criticisms of medical education outlined above remain valid; being based on a mechanistic concept of disease and of medical intervention, it begins with consideration of the structure and function of the body, continues with discussion of disease processes and ends with clinical experience of selected hospital patients. In such circumstances it is very difficult to convey that medicine has a vital contribution to the non-personal and behavioural influences which are the main determinants of ill health, and that the care of patients who are permanently handicapped or in terminal illness is as much part of the medical responsibility as investigation and treatment of acute disease.

5. It was suggested above that there is need for medical specialists who devote themselves wholly to environmental medicine. Such specialists cannot be expected to emerge unless the subject is presented adequately when they are undergraduates. A recent survey of medical schools in the United Kingdom showed that only 15 of 25 schools gave any formal instruction in occupational health, the part of the field that has had most attention in medical education, and the time allowed was generally small: less than six hours in 8 of the 15 schools which included some teaching.

THE IMAGE OF MEDICINE PROJECTED AT THE TEACHING CENTRE

But the really potent influence on students, and through them on the subsequent operation of health services, is neither the selection procedures of medical schools nor the design of medical curricula; it is the image of medicine which emerges from the range of activities and interests of the teaching centre.

It is not difficult to understand how the restriction of the work of teaching hospitals came about; it resulted from grafting the concept of scientific medicine on to the tradition of the voluntary hospitals.

From the time of their rebirth under secular auspices in the eighteenth century the large voluntary hospitals attempted to limit their work to short-term remediable cases which were of greatest interest to the medical staff and were said to make the best use of their resources. Thus they excluded the majority of patients who had to be cared for in separate voluntary hospitals (for example, for women and children) or in public institutions (for the infectious, the mentally ill, and the destitute).

It is important to recognize that the work of voluntary hospitals was not designed to meet the needs of medical education; on the contrary, medical education had to conform to the established traditions of the hospitals. In Britain at the end of the eighteenth century the training of doctors was still mainly in private profit-making schools and there were nineteen different corporations with the power to examine and license medical practitioners. Only three London hospitals (St Bartholomew's, the United Hospitals– St Thomas's and Guy's– and the London) had medical schools attached to them. The association between medical education and voluntary hospitals did not develop rapidly until the nineteenth century, when the College of Surgeons and the Society of Apothecaries included hospital work among requirements from candidates for their examinations. By this time the lines of interest of some of the major hospitals had been drawn for more than a hundred years.

Moreover there was no disposition on the part of teachers to challenge the limited spectrum of interests at the hospitals, for they were themselves the consultants, or the heirs of the consultants, who had been largely responsible for restricting their work. Indeed the opportunity to have students who would later refer patients was one of the attractions of hospital appointments, and it would have been surprising indeed if the teaching commitment had led consultants to challenge the premises on which their own work was based. It has scarcely done so a hundred and fifty years later when there is less excuse for failure to recognize the limitations of the earlier tradition.

Eventually, of course, some hospitals were founded as teaching hospitals (University College Hospital, for example, in 1828). But by this time the idea of the acute general hospital as the focus of medical education was deeply rooted, and the role of the new hospitals established for teaching did not differ significantly from that of the existing hospitals to which teaching responsibilities were added later. In this way medical education became based on institutions which attempted to exclude (among other patients) the destitute and the infectious, at a time when poverty was widespread and infection the predominant cause of death. Preoccupied with his own interests, the consultant teacher had apparently not noticed that he had removed from the attention of the student the most formidable medical problems of his day. In doing so he also determined the direction of medical education and the scope of the work of the teaching centre for more than a century.

The exclusive character of the work of the teaching centre was further accentuated by the trend towards scientific medicine on which the Flexner Report had so great an influence. Flexner suggested that 'medical education must be conceived as primarily the effort to train students in the intellectual technique of inductive science', a view which would be widely endorsed in academic circles today. He recognized that 'education in science is somewhat different from the aquisition of information and the control of mechanism; it concerns itself fundamentally with habituation to method'. In a very significant passage he went on to say: 'Knowledge is indeed necessary, inasmuch as scientific method does not operate in a vacuum. A selection must therefore be made, and, unless the teacher is perverse, it will be made with general, *though by no means uniform*, reference to the objects of professional training' (italics inserted).

These ideas have influenced the thinking of a generation. Whether justly or not, they have been interpreted to strengthen the case for selectiveness. If a student is encouraged to think clearly and critically, if he learns (for example) to understand the inflammatory process, to examine the central nervous system, and to interpret an electrocardiograph and X-ray, he can apply his knowledge and methods in the very varied circumstances in which he may find himself after qualification, and for which in any case it would be impossible for medical education to prepare him in detail. From this it is concluded that the exhibition of a wide range of patients and services to students is a secondary consideration; indeed experience of the scientific method can be acquired more readily from a small number of patients carefully selected and

3. McKeown, T., *Medicine in Modern Society* (London: George Allen and Unwin Ltd, 1965), pp. 213–21.

fully investigated. And if some or all of these patients are the focus of the research interests of the clinical teacher, this can only make the instruction more stimulating and effective than otherwise it would be.

The effects of the traditions of the teaching hospitals on medical education have been profound. A medical service can be no more enlightened than the minds of the doctors who provide it, and the intellectual shutters are never again so widely open as during the period of training. Inevitably students acquire their concept of practice from the example provided by their teachers, and they leave the hospital aspiring to engage in the work they saw when training.

It is for this reason that the isolation of teaching from some of the major health problems is so serious. A centre which excludes the mentally ill, the subnormal, and many of the aged sick cannot be expected to provide doctors who will care for them; and even the token admission of a few of these patients does not convey the idea that these are the largest and most formidable problems by which medicine is now confronted. It is not possible to staff the major services unless the full range of problems and methods is displayed at the teaching centre where the work and interests of the future doctor are determined.

The effects of the restrictions are even more grotesque in developing countries, where the western model has been adopted with little modification, and without regard for the vastly different problems and resources. Teaching hospitals are usually remote from the rural areas where most people live and the health needs are greatest. Indeed it is one of the anomalies of medical education that, with its focus on disease mechanisms rather than disease origins, it aspires to a concept of practice which is uniform and presupposes the existence of selected patients and the availability of unlimited resources.

I have discussed elsewhere the changes needed to correct the deficiencies.[3] Ideally the teaching centre should accept responsibility for all medical services for the population of a defined area, or where this is not possible, for all hospital services and a close association with domiciliary and other health and related social services.

TRAINING OF OTHER HEALTH WORKERS

There is a further point which concerns the relation between the trainings of medical and other health workers. It is perhaps not too fanciful to imagine that in this context history might be divided into three periods: the first, ending in 1858, when major issues divided the various classes of medical workers: physicians, surgeons, and apothecaries; the second, from the passing of the First Medical Act (in 1858) to the present day, when doctors were a uniform profession, dominant in the health scene and with no major problems in their relation to one another or to other workers; and a third period which we have now entered, when important issues arise concerning the respective roles of medicine and other health professions. It is significant that in the present period the concept of a uniform medical profession is also being eroded, by the introduction (particularly in the United States) of a substantial element of elective work in medical education. Doctors are no longer identical at the time they take their medical qualification, but have already established in a preliminary way their roles as specialists. It is difficult to be confident about the long-term effects of this trend, for good or ill. But what should be noted is that the relation of doctors to nurses, social workers, hygienists, indeed to all the major groups in the health field, becomes very much an open question when the identity of the physician himself is no longer so clearly defined.

12

Medical Research

In his poem, based on the myth of Leda and the Swan, Yeats asked whether the girl, seduced by the transformed god, 'put on his knowledge with his power'.[1] The same question when inverted might be asked about medicine today: Did it put on its power with its knowledge? However, it is one of the charms of the fable that it is open to more than one interpretation, so I must avoid misunderstanding by stating the issue more precisely: Are the improvements in health with which medicine is commonly credited determined essentially by medical science, or are they due largely to fortuitous changes in which bio-medical research has played little part?

Most scientists, certainly most medical scientists, are in no doubt about the answer. Since the eighteenth century health has been transformed; since the nineteenth century medical knowledge has greatly increased; and in the twentieth century there have been remarkable advances in technology. These events are assumed to be causally related, the improvement in health being attributed to the growth of knowledge, and the new knowledge, essentially, to medical research. From this interpretation of the past hopes are projected into the future; what science is believed to have done is thought to give grounds for confidence in what science can be expected to do. Yesterday the decline of the infections, tomorrow control of cancer and mental illness. Indeed as Burnet has reminded us, medical research workers hold a unique place among scientists largely because their work is believed to contribute powerfully to the saving of human life.[2]

Any questioning of these views can be counted on to provoke an immediate and sharp response. In his book *Genes, Dreams and Realities*,

1. 'So mastered by the brute blood of the air, Did she put on his knowledge with his power?'
2. Burnett, Sir Macfarlane, *Genes, Dreams and Realities* (Aylesbury, Bucks: Medical and Technical Publishing Co. Ltd, 1971), p. 226.

156

Burnet concluded that 'the contribution of laboratory science has virtually come to an end' and 'almost none of modern basic research in the medical sciences has any direct bearing on the prevention of disease or on the improvement of medical care'.[3] One reviewer reacted to these heresies like a devout clergyman who has heard his bishop express doubts about the divinity of Christ. Burnet was accused not merely of scientific error, but even more seriously, of lacking faith in the potential of science.

And finally the contribution to medicine that can be expected from laboratory research as a whole. The major medical problems now facing advanced societies are indeed difficult ones; no one expects rapid or dramatic solutions (although they may turn up, as they have so often done before, in the most unexpected ways). But one can be sure of one thing; solutions will not come without laboratory research. If society wants solutions to current medical problems (and it does), then it is laboratory research that it must support. There are no alternatives.[4]

It is perhaps not stretching the clerical analogy too far to suggest that this passage is concerned with faith as well as fact: 'Believe or ye are lost', and in the last despairing sentence, 'Believe and ye may still be lost.'

But it would be wrong to imply that medical scientists' estimate of the contribution of their work is attributable largely to emotion; many believe that they have assessed health problems accurately when they say that the ability to prevent sickness and premature death is based on knowledge derived from laboratory research, often of the pure variety. When considering the contribution of technology to medicine Thomas wrote: 'If I were a policy-maker, interested in saving money for health care over the long haul, I would regard it as an act of high prudence to give high priority to a lot more basic research in biologic science.'[5] And in a discussion of pure and applied research Medawar concluded: 'We encourage pure research in these situations because we know no other way to go about it. If we knew of a direct pathway leading to the solution of the clinical problem of rheumatoid arthritis, can anyone seriously believe that we should not take it?'[6]

3. Burnet, op. cit., p. 218.
4. Harris, Henry, *British Medical Journal*, 3 (1971), p. 712.
5. Thomas, L., *The Lives of a Cell* (Toronto, New York, London: Bantam Books, Inc., 1975), p. 41.
6. Medawar, P. B., *The Art of the Soluble* (Great Britain: Pelican Books, 1969), p. 137.

I believe that the thinking of those who take this view of the contribution of medical research is influenced by the Cartesian model; in concluding that improvements in health are derived exclusively from understanding of the structure and function of the body and of the disease processes that affect it they are carrying over to living things principles which have been applied successfully to inanimate matter. But they would long since have rejected this model if it were thought to be seriously inconsistent with experience. The fact that they have not done so indicates that they believe the decline of infectious disease, the main reason for the improvement in health, was due essentially to the increased knowledge provided by medical science. To evaluate this conclusion we must examine closely the contribution of science and technology to the main influences, nutritional, environmental, behavioural, and medical, which were responsible for the reduction of infectious deaths.

SCIENCE, TECHNOLOGY, AND HEALTH

In assessing the impact of science and technology it will be desirable to distinguish clearly between the following:

1. Measures which, although scientific in character, owed little if anything to professional science. I am thinking, for example, of manuring of land by farmers and limitation of family size by parents.

2. Measures derived from investigations of a relatively simple epidemiological kind. I refer to the introduction of environmental improvements before the nature of infectious disease was understood, as a result of observations on living conditions and health.

3. Non-medical science and technology which extended the measures referred to under 1: for example, chemical fertilizers, insecticides, and herbicides in agriculture, and engineering technology which contributed to control of the environment.

4. Biomedical research which extended non-personal measures. Perhaps the best example is the understanding of the nature of infectious disease which led to improvements in hygiene of water and food.

5. Biomedical research which resulted in immunization and treatment.

In the present context it will be particularly interesting to distinguish the contribution of medical science (4 and 5) from that of other influences (1, 2, and 3); and within medical science, to see the extent to which its impact was through personal measures (immunization and therapy) as distinct from non-personal measures such as hygiene and better food. For the application of the Cartesian model to the problems of human health might be interpreted in either of two ways. It might be taken to mean that health depended on understanding of the body and disease processes, that is on the significance of 4. Or, on a stricter interpretation of the concept, it might be interpreted to mean that health was determined by control of the body as a machine, that is by the personal measures of immunization and therapy referred to under 5.

I shall consider briefly the nature of the more important developments before commenting on their scientific character.

NUTRITION

The improvement in nutrition was due initially to advances in agriculture which spread throughout the western world from about the end of the seventeenth century. The following developments were particularly important to the production and distribution of food.

(*a*) Improvement in organization, particularly enclosure of land which encouraged more efficient farming.

(*b*) Advances in farming practice, which included conservation of fertility, crop rotation, seed production, winter feeding, minor improvements in farm implements and, notably, the introduction of root crops, particularly the potato and, in warm climates, maize.

(*c*) Improvements in transport, initially by navigable rivers and roads but later by canals.

These were the critical advances in the eighteenth and nineteenth centuries, and they led to a large increase in food production. Hutchinson attached particular importance to the restoration of fertility through manuring,[7] and Langer assembled impressive evidence for the significance of root crops, introduced from the New World in the seventeenth century.[8] Whatever the relative importance of the different advances there is no doubt that they resulted from more intensive and systematic use of traditional farming methods rather than the introduction of new ones. From the second half of the nineteenth century, however, agricultural output was increased further by mechanization, chemical fertilizers and later, insecticides and herbicides.

7. Hutchinson, J., 'Land and human populations', *The Advancement of Science*, **23** (1966), 241.

8. Langer, W. L., 'American foods and Europe's population growth, 1750–1850', *Journal of Social History*, Winter Number (1975), p. 51.

HYGIENE

The question whether the environmental measures developed in the nineteenth century were initially of a scientific kind is an intriguing one. It might be argued that they were not, on the grounds that Chadwick, the most effective advocate of reform, did not accept the explanation for their success suggested by the work of Pasteur: that micro-organisms were the cause of infectious diseases. However, the ideas which led Chadwick and his colleagues to the conclusion that the environment was an important source of illness had been evolving over more than a century. As early as 1719, when plague appeared again in southern Europe, Richard Meade suggested not only more stringent application of traditional measures (isolation and quarantine) but also much wider improvements in the community: better housing, cleanliness, ventilation, disinfection, and control of nuisances. A little later there were notable investigations of the association between living conditions and disease, by Pringle in the army, Lind in the navy, and Howard in his poignant journey through English prisons in the winter of 1773. Two practical demonstrations of the feasibility of control of disease by environmental measures were the observations that scurvy could be prevented by eating fresh fruit, and that the colic which was endemic in Devon was attributable to lead poisoning. But perhaps the most significant inquiry was largely the work of Chadwick, who published in 1842 his *Report on the Sanitary Conditions of the Labouring Population of Great Britain*. This document examined the relation between environmental conditions and ill-health. By later standards much of the evidence was deficient; nevertheless it was essentially of an epidemiological kind which today, in spite of methodological reservations, we should unhesitatingly regard as scientific.

The effectiveness of hygienic measures was greatly extended from the time when Pasteur established the bacterial origin of infectious diseases. Microbiology was of course the source of preventive and therapeutic measures applied to the individual; but it also contributed powerfully to advances in hygiene which were even more important, for example by showing how infection is spread, and making it possible to identify specific diseases, including their unsuspected presence in 'carriers'.

REPRODUCTIVE BEHAVIOUR

There were no specific biological or other scientific developments behind the modification of reproductive behaviour which led to the decline of the birth-rate. It might, perhaps, be said that the work of Malthus and, less directly, of Darwin had drawn attention to the importance of control of numbers; but by 1870 when the birth-rate began to decline in England and Wales, this knowledge can have reached only a small and selected segment of the population. Moreover, in France the fall of the birth-rate began much earlier, and indeed was already evident at the end of eighteenth century when Malthus was writing. It therefore seems permissible to conclude that in the beginning the limitation of numbers was due, not to any identifiable scientific advance, but to the fact that large numbers of people had reached the conclusion that the lives of their families would be improved if they restricted the number of children. I shall not attempt to speculate on whether this simple observation was in some sense scientific; what is not in doubt is that methods of control of reproduction were later extended by science, although their contribution in practice is still something of an open question.

IMMUNIZATION AND THERAPY

Many medical scientists believe that the control of bacterial infections is based on knowledge of infectious diseases derived from basic research and applied largely, although by no means exclusively, through immunization and therapy. In Chapter 6 I arrived at quite a different conclusion: that these measures had little effect on the death-rate before 1935 and since that time have been less important than other influences. Diphtheria was the only *common* infection in which a specific measure, immunization, may have been the main reason for its decline; in the other common ones (tuberculosis, pneumonia, measles, whooping cough and scarlet fever) mortality had fallen to a relatively low level before effective medical intervention was possible. The diseases (smallpox, syphilis, poliomyelitis, and tetanus) in which specific measures are generally regarded as the main reason for their decline, taken singly or collectively made only a small contribution to the total reduction of infectious deaths.

This appraisal suggests that the modern improvement in health was initiated and carried quite a long way with little contribution from science and technology, except for the epidemiological investigations of environmental conditions in the eighteenth and early nineteenth centuries. This was true of the increase in food production, the beginning of hygienic measures and control of numbers. These advances resulted from simple but fundamental observations on everyday life: conservation of fertility increased agricultural output; hygienic measures prevented infectious diseases; and limitation of the number of births improved the conditions of life for parents and their children.

However, from the second half of the nineteenth century the original steps were extended by scientific developments of a non-personal kind (3 and 4 above). Some of these (for example improved transport, chemical fertilizers and mechanization in agriculture, technology in distribution of water and disposal of sewage, and refrigeration in transportation of food) owed little to biomedical science and would have been introduced even if no health interests were involved. But for extension and refinement of methods of preventing the spread of infectious diseases we are indebted to medical science and particularly to laboratory research.

Since this interpretation of the contribution of science in the past has a considerable bearing on the approach to research in the future, it is important to consider a possible ground for reservation. Is it conceivable that things might have been quite different, that it was an accident of history that agricultural and other advances preceded effective medical intervention, and had the latter been available earlier its impact on mortality would have been more impressive?

The effect of immunization and therapy on a population which is underfed and heavily exposed to infection is something of an open question; so far as it goes, experience of the World Health Organization in developing countries suggests that it is questionable whether infectious disease can be controlled by vaccination in a malnourished population. But if there is doubt about the effectiveness of medical measures in the absence of advances in nutrition and hygiene, there is none about the effectiveness of advances in nutrition and hygiene in the absence of medical measures. Experience of the last two centuries indicates that infectious deaths fell to a small fraction of their earlier level without medical intervention, and suggests that had none been available they would have continued to decline, if not so rapidly in some diseases.

Those who look mainly to laboratory research for the solution of health problems do so under some misapprehensions about its achievements in the past. They underestimate the part that has been played by a rising standard of living and the accompanying advance in literacy, and they overestimate the contribution of laboratory medicine, particularly as applied through immunization and therapy. However, they are not mistaken in regarding as important the increased understanding of disease processes which resulted from biomedical science, taking that term to include both laboratory and epidemiological research.

The tendency to overestimate the significance of laboratory investigation is well illustrated by a recent assessment of the contribution of basic and applied research to 'lifesaving advances' in cardiovascular and pulmonary diseases.[9] The advances examined were open-heart surgery, blood vessel surgery, treatment of hypertension, management of coronary artery disease, prevention of poliomyelitis, chemotherapy of tuberculosis and acute rheumatic fever, cardiac resuscitation and cardiac pacemakers, oral diuretics (for treatment of high blood pressure or of congestive heart failure), intensive care units, and new diagnostic methods. The authors were able to show that these advances relied largely on work which 'was not clinically oriented at the time it was done', and they concluded 'that a generous portion of the nation's biomedical research dollars should be used to identify and then to provide long-term support for creative scientists whose main goal is to learn how living organisms function, without regard to the immediate relation of their research to specific human diseases'.

In the present context what is remarkable is not the suggestion that fundamental research is indispensable, but the selection of advances on which this conclusion is based. Of the ten listed above, one is concerned with methods, and is therefore only a means to a therapeutic end. Two others refer to a large contribution to a relatively small problem (prevention of poliomyelitis) or to small contributions to large problems (chemotherapy of tuberculosis and acute rheumatic fever). The rest are all examples of what Thomas describes as 'halfway technology . . . the kinds of things that must be done after the fact, in efforts to compensate for the incapacitating effects of certain diseases whose course one is unable to do very much about'.[10] Such measures may prolong life for a few years; but they do not prevent the diseases, nor do they restore the patient to a life of normal duration and quality.

The distinction between prolonging life for a limited period and the solution of a major disease problem may also be illustrated by reference to diabetes. The discovery of insulin is regarded as one of the landmarks in the history of medical research and it is sometimes said that 'insulin

9. Comroe (Jr), J. H., and Dripps, R. D., 'Scientific basis for the support of biomedical science', *Science*, **192** (1976), 105.

10. Thomas, L., *The Lives of a Cell* (Toronto, New York, London: Bantam Books, Inc., 1975), p. 37.

enables diabetics to live as long as other persons and to have as many children'.[11] Certainly it is true that insulin has prolonged many lives; nevertheless in England and Wales diabetes was given as the primary cause of 5,127 deaths (nearly 1 per cent of all deaths) in 1973, and it must also have been entered as a secondary cause in many more. And while diabetics who would formerly have been sterile now have normal children, the pregnancy of a diabetic woman is still a source of anxiety; even in the best hospitals, perinatal mortality is close to 10 per cent, about five times the rate in non-diabetic mothers.[12] It is also doubtful whether treatment can control the secondary complications of the disease: for example cataract, neuropathy, and vascular disease.[13] Clearly, although the multiple problems which arise from diabetes have been greatly alleviated by insulin, they have by no means been solved.

In making our cheerful assessments of the results of research whose goal 'is to learn how living organisms function', we have been looking through a lens of high power at a small segment of a large field. Within that segment the advances from laboratory science have of course been very valuable; but over the whole range of disease problems their contribution was limited, and it would have been seen to be limited if human health had not been transformed in the same period by other influences. The key to the main direction of medical research in the future lies in close appraisal of these influences.

In Chapter 6 I concluded that in order of importance the determinants of health were nutritional, environmental, and behavioural in the past, and will probably be behavioural, environmental, and nutritional in the future, at least in developed countries. The theoretical grounds for their effectiveness were outlined in Chapter 2. During his evolution man, like other living things, was exposed to rigorous natural selection which restricted disease determined irreversibly at fertilization to a low frequency. Most diseases and disabilities are therefore due to environmental influences operating on variable genetic material, and the solution of disease problems depends essentially on the removal or modification of the deleterious agents.

On this interpretation of common diseases, a full understanding of

11. Dubos, R., *Man, Medicine and Environment* (London: Pall Mall Press, 1968), p. 85.

12. Leading article, *British Medical Journal*, **2** (1976), 267.

13. Butterfield, W. J. H., 'Diabetes mellitus', in *Screening in Medical Care* (London, New York, Toronto: Oxford University Press for the Nuffield Provincial Hospitals Trust, 1968), p. 76.

disease processes is often unnecessary for their control. The decline of infectious deaths preceded by more than a hundred years the discovery of micro-organisms; withdrawal of thalidomide and avoidance of exposure to rubella in pregnancy prevented the associated malformations without knowledge of teratogenesis; and cessation of smoking by doctors lowered the incidence of cancer of the lung in spite of very incomplete information about the natural history of the disease and the mechanism of carcinogenesis.

The grounds for reservations concerning the conventional view of health problems – that their solution depends on knowledge of disease acquired by laboratory research and applied mainly through medical intervention – are therefore both pragmatic and conceptual. This explanation is not in accord with past experience; nor is it consistent with interpretation of the origins of disease.

The conclusion that a detailed knowledge of mechanisms is often not essential for the solution of biological problems is confirmed by experience of everyday life. One of the best sires at stud is a horse called *Vaguely Noble*, whose reputation is based on the observations that he was himself a great racehorse and that he has already sired some very fast offspring, including *Pawneese* (the leading 3-year-old in Europe, unbeaten to 1976) and the great French filly, *Dahlia*. This success owes nothing to unravelling of the genetic code or even to Mendelism or Darwinism, but is based on breeding practices that have been in use since plants and animals were first domesticated ten thousand years ago. . . . Some of the finest wines ever made, for example La Tâche, La Romanée, and La Romanée-Conti, are produced without assistance from laboratory science in a few acres of Burgundy, by combining knowledge of soil, sun, wind, and rain, with traditions of wine-making that have been perfected with pride and affection, and passed from father to son and from nobleman to peasant for generations. Does anyone imagine that within the foreseeable future faster racehorses could be bred by modifications of gene structure, or that wines of equal or greater subtlety could be manufactured by substituting chemical and biological methods for the traditional viniculture?

The problems which would arise in dealing with common diseases by intervention at the molecular or cellular level are no less formidable. Indeed since piano playing, to take another example, involves only two variables, interval and pressure, technically the replacement of Kempff's Beethoven and Rubinstein's Chopin by mechanically produced sound would be hardly more than a five-finger exercise, if compared with the difficulties of preventing mental subnormality, cancer, or heart disease by control of genes.

Contrary to what is generally believed, the most fundamental issue confronting medical science is not the solution of one or more of the unsolved biomedical problems: it is evaluation of two approaches to the control of disease, one through an understanding of mechanisms and the other through a knowledge of origins. And as both approaches are needed, what is required is a decision about the distribution of effort between them and, if possible, identification of the circumstances in which each is likely to be rewarding.

Since epidemiologists are concerned particularly with disease origins and clinicians and laboratory investigators with mechanisms, it may be thought that what is in question is the respective roles of epidemiology and other kinds of research. However, this way of looking at the matter is misleading. The discovery of micro-organisms in the laboratory contributed enormously to control of the origins of infectious diseases; and epidemiological investigations of the distribution of blood pressure in the general population were necessary for an understanding of the nature of essential hypertension. The emphasis therefore should be on disease origins and mechanisms, each investigated by the methods – population, clinical, experimental – that seem appropriate to the problem in hand.

There is not much room for disagreement about the contribution of these approaches in the past. Health advanced because of the decline of the infections; and the infections declined mainly because of modification of the conditions which led to them. This conclusion is unaffected by well-founded doubts about the reliability of data (based on certification of cause of death) for individual diseases, and by recognition that understanding of disease mechanisms has made it possible to treat a number of conditions. No knowledgeable person is likely to dispute that we owe the vast increase in expectation of life and reduction of associated morbidity mainly to changes which occurred before effective clinical intervention was possible.

We are on less certain ground when we turn from interpretation of the past to speculation about the future. The infections declined largely because of removal of the ill-effects of poverty, and the non-communicable diseases which have replaced them are evidently not responsive to the same changes, otherwise they would not be there. How then are we to decide in what circumstances each of the main lines of enquiry is likely to be successful?

Before trying to answer this question I must refer briefly to the residual disease problems in developed countries. They are often assessed by analysis of causes of death at all ages. Treated in this way they include deaths (the majority) at the end of a normal expectation of life, which have presumably been determined at fertilization, as well as premature deaths not so determined which are in principle preventable. In so far as prevention of death is a goal of medical science, it is only the latter which are relevant. As the genetically determined expectation of life (for those not congenitally handicapped) is about eighty years, it would be better to base the analysis of preventable deaths on deaths at an earlier age, say before seventy. These would inevitably include some deaths which were genetically determined, just as they would exclude some later deaths which were not. They would, however, provide a much better basis for assessment of the tasks of medical science than deaths at all ages.

I suggest that the approaches needed to the residual disease problems can be clarified by consideration of the four-fold classification of diseases outlined in Chapter 7: relatively intractable; preventable, associated with poverty; preventable, associated with affluence; and potentially preventable, not known to be related to poverty or affluence.

RELATIVELY INTRACTABLE

The diseases in this class comprise genetic diseases (single-gene disorders and chromosomal aberrations), some polygenic conditions determined at fertilization, and diseases not so determined in which the environmental influences are prenatal. While it is possible that some in the last group may be due to influences which can be identified and controlled (such as thalidomide and rubella), there are so far no grounds for thinking that this will be the case with most of the common congenital conditions.

In principle three approaches are possible to congenital disease (whether determined at fertilization or *in utero*): prevention of conception; recognition during pregnancy and elimination by abortion; and treatment after birth.

On present knowledge we have no grounds for optimism about the possibility of preventing conception by identification of parents likely

168 *The Role of Medicine*

to have affected children. Penrose estimated that avoidance of conception by subnormal parents would not have a large effect on the frequency of mental subnormality in the general population.[14] The conclusion seems inescapable that the most promising approach to the control of serious congenital diseases which can be neither prevented nor successfully treated is identification during pregnancy and removal by abortion. Having regard to the size and intractability of the problems, there are few more important tasks for medical research than the study of methods of recognizing abnormal embryos or foetuses early in pregnancy.

This is not to suggest that there should be no further interest in other lines of investigation. Prevention of rhesus haemolytic diseases was referred to earlier as an example of prevention, and correction of some cardiac malformations by surgery as an example of successful treatment. Nevertheless, within the foreseeable future it would be unrealistic to expect prevention or treatment to provide a solution of the most formidable congenital problems.

Most polygenic conditions determined at fertilization are manifested in late life: for example, sensory defects, limitation of mobility, and various disabilities associated with deficient blood supply. Since these abnormalities may occur at the end of a long and healthy life, prevention of the birth of those likely to be affected is not a recommendable aim. The only possible approach is by clinical intervention, which has been very successful in some cases, for example in the treatment of eye conditions or replacement of an arthritic hip.

However, the main conclusion to be drawn is that with the possible exception of some determined *in utero*, the diseases referred to as relatively intractable are unlikely to be controlled by modifying their origins, and must be approached by understanding their mechanisms. This indeed is the field which uniquely requires the traditional laboratory and clinical approach, and the more successful post-natal measures are in dealing with preventable conditions, the more important the residual prenatal problems will be seen to be.

PREVENTABLE, ASSOCIATED WITH POVERTY

The predominant health problems of the world are still those associated with poverty (Chapter 7), particularly the infectious diseases of developing countries whose control requires the application of well-tried

14. Penrose, L. S., *The Biology of Mental Defect* (London: Sidgwick and Jackson Ltd, 1963), p. 288.

methods directed at disease origins: provision of food; improvements in hygiene; limitation of numbers; and, in tropical countries, control of vectors. However, there are some infections (malaria, yellow fever, measles, tuberculosis, tetanus, etc.) in which clinical measures based on an understanding of disease mechanisms also have an important part to play.

The rate of advance is determined largely by the wealth of a country, and to this extent the problems are economic rather than medical. However, a good deal also depends on the wise use of resources available for health purposes, and here the critical influence of food and hygiene should be recognized. With diseases such as malaria and schistosomiasis the difficulties are compounded by the problem of controlling the vectors – the mosquito and the snail – which so far have been able to resist all the measures directed against them. It is an open question whether the most successful approach will be an attack on the vector or parasite, or an improvement in the defences of the human host. In view of the uncertainty, the prudent decision is to explore all three possibilities.

Many problems of non-communicable disease and disability in developed countries are also related to poverty, and again their solution turns largely on the resources available. For example, if the costs were not prohibitive it would be possible greatly to reduce the frequency of domestic, industrial and traffic accidents, to eliminate many toxic and other hazards in industry, and to speed up improvements in the general environment, for example by more rigorous control of pollution of lakes, rivers and seas as well as the atmosphere.

In relation to medical research the chief points to be noted about the diseases associated with poverty are: that for the world as a whole they are still predominant; that many of the measures required are already known and are largely, although by no means entirely, concerned with disease origins; that improvement is restricted by lack of resources (and to that extent the problems are economic); that there are still important unsolved problems related to both origins and mechanisms (as in diseases such as malaria and schistosomiasis).

PREVENTABLE, ASSOCIATED WITH AFFLUENCE

If attention is restricted to developed countries, the predominant health problems are those related to an excess rather than to a deficiency of resources. The grounds for this conclusion were discussed in Chapter 7

and we are concerned here only with its significance for medical research. Two questions which arise are: which diseases should be included
in this class; and are they more likely to be controlled by modification
of behaviour or by intervention in disease processes?

The diseases which might be considered fall into three groups. In the
first there are those attributable to smoking, drugs, alcohol, and perhaps
excessive food intake, in which there is no doubt about the nature of
the influence or of the benefits which would follow from its withdrawal.

The second group comprises conditions in which the evidence is
suggestive but incomplete, as in the case of the effects of insufficient
fibre in the diet or of the links between fats and lack of exercise
and coronary artery disease. There is, I suggest, an important,
methodological point which should be noted when environmental influences are multiple. The experiment on *Drosophila* referred to in
Chapter 2 shows the difficulty of partitioning variance between nature
and nurture, because their relative contributions are not constant over
more than a narrow environmental range. There is good reason to
think that the contributions of different environmental influences also
vary in relation to the environment. For example, the ill-effects of
asbestos are very much greater in smokers than non-smokers. This variation no doubt accounts for some of the difficulty in establishing the
effects of multiple environmental influences.

There is a third group of diseases in which it seems probable that
behavioural influences are important but in which the evidence is even
less complete. I am thinking particularly of many types of mental illness,
including the psychoses as well as the neuroses and psychosomatic conditions.

For the purposes of the present discussion I shall restrict the diseases
classified as 'preventable, associated with affluence' to the first two
groups in which the evidence of behavioural influences is at or near the
level at which action might be taken to modify them.

The question remains whether modification of behaviour or intervention in disease processes offers the best approach. Here one can only
express a personal view. I believe that the solution or partial solution
of the problems of lung cancer, coronary artery disease, chronic bronchitis and peripheral vascular disease is more likely to come from avoidance of smoking than from medical treatment. However, the time scale
is important: for substantial changes in smoking habits we should be
thinking in decades rather than years, and in the meantime any advance

that can be made in the treatment of these conditions will be greatly needed. Extending the same thinking, I conclude that for a solution of the predominant behavioural problems of our time we should be searching mainly for ways of controlling disease origins, while not neglecting anything that can be applied from increased knowledge of disease mechanisms.

POTENTIALLY PREVENTABLE, NOT KNOWN TO BE RELATED TO POVERTY OR AFFLUENCE

The discussion so far of the two approaches to medical research can be summarized as follows. The solution to the predominant health problems of the past, and also of the present when developing countries are included, depended mainly on an attack on disease origins associated with poverty. When attention is restricted to technologically advanced countries, the predominant residual problems are determined by behaviour, so that again the control of disease origins seems to be the more promising approach. But increasingly as poverty is relieved and people learn to behave themselves, the hard core of diseases which remain will be those determined at fertilization or arising during prenatal life. The solution of such problems by prevention, abortion or treatment can be achieved only by increased knowledge of disease mechanisms.

However, this brief summary leaves out of account a fourth class of diseases which are in principle preventable – there is no reason to believe they are determined at fertilization – but about which not enough is known to enable us to judge the nature of the environmental influences concerned. A number of conditions are on the borderline, but I suggest that most mental illnesses fall into this class, whereas most cancers are in the preceding one.

These are the diseases over which opinion about the best approach will be most widely divided, so what follows can be no more than a personal judgement.

Infectious diseases. There are a number of infections which have not responded to improvements in the standard of living and whose distribution is little influenced by social class. I am thinking particularly of airborne diseases such as influenza and the common cold, but also of many acute gastro-intestinal infections. It is difficult to see how such diseases can be prevented by controlling their origins or transmission, and intervention by immunization or treatment seems the only feasible approach. For this we require increased knowledge of the disease mechanisms. The position is of course quite different for venereal infections, which are determined by sexual behaviour.

Mental illness. Mental illness presents one of the most serious challenges to medical research: there is little evidence of success in the past, for with the exception of the form due to an infection (syphilis of the central nervous system), there has been no response to the influences which have brought about the decline of physical (mainly infectious) diseases. But the slow rate of progress has at least the excuse that the problems are inherently difficult; it is a fair guess that if all the Nobel prize-winners of this century had worked in psychiatry, the subject would have advanced only a little less slowly and none of them would have received the prize.

But in what direction should we be looking? During man's evolution, natural selection must have restricted the frequency of genetically determined mental illness to a low level. The common diseases such as mental subnormality and the psychoses are therefore not established irreversibly at fertilization, but are due to influences acting on variable genetic material. Operationally the important consideration is not the nature of the genetic component or the balance sheet of nature and nurture; it is the feasibility of identifying and controlling the environmental influences.

In the case of mental subnormality these influences are usually, although not invariably, prenatal; in the case of the psychoses and psychoneuroses, it seems reasonable to believe as a working hypothesis that they are mainly post-natal. And just as we think of agents entering the nose and mouth as likely to be important in respiratory and digestive diseases, so we should look to behavioural influences as the probable source of most disorders of behaviour.

Unfortunately Freudian psychology, which might have been expected to lead in this direction, from this point of view at least has been a disappointment. Therapeutically it has merely conferred a secular blessing on the practice of confession, and with its emphasis on therapy it has not led to the search for influences which might be modified or removed. What are needed are not so much recollections of how parents treated their children in the distant past, as observations on how they treat them in the present.

But it is by no means certain that the conventional approach, even of epidemiology, will be successful when applied to the study of behaviour. Let us imagine a line drawn from Jesus Christ to Dr Gallup and passing through such eminent investigators of the human condition as Karl Marx, Max Weber, the Webbs, and Dr Kinsey. While there might be differences of opinion about the order of names, I think it would be generally agreed that from Christ to Gallup the issues become pettier and the scope for research, particularly of a numerical kind, becomes greater. When Christ said 'he that findeth his life shall lose it', and La Rochefoucauld 'that it is easier to generalize about mankind than to understand any one man', perceptive people recognize that they were making profound observations on the human condition. Yet their conclusions were not the result of scientific inquiry and, once made, no science was needed to validate them.

The conclusion to be drawn is that the solution, however distant, of a psychiatric problem such as schizophrenia may come, not from treatment of the established disorder by biochemical or other methods, but, as in the case of all other major diseases which have so far been controlled, by removal of the influences which led to the abnormality. If so, the main emphasis of medical research should be on identifying those influences, by observing and reflecting carefully on the history of schizophrenics and their families, by comparing them with non-affected families, and by examining the experience of the disease in different populations and sections of populations. This is of course the approach of the epidemiologist; but he will need even more inspiration than in the study of physical illness. In general, he should proceed like Christ rather than Gallup, suspecting the answer before starting to look for it, and using subsequent research to provide an opportunity for his hunches to be proved wrong.

Other diseases. There remain a number of physical illnesses whose aetiology is still obscure: for example, some cancers, rheumatoid arthritis, osteoarthritis and multiple sclerosis. How are we to decide in such cases which of the two main lines of investigation is likely to be most successful?

I suggest that a disease whose incidence varies substantially in different populations or population subgroups is more likely to be controlled by modifying the conditions that lead to it. This has been true of nearly all the disease problems that could be said to have been solved hitherto, and it seems reasonable to accept it as a working hypothesis until there are some obvious exceptions. Infections in which immunization and treatment are effective might be mentioned, but with the possible exception of poliomyelitis there is none in which we could say confidently that the conditions which led to them were not profoundly altered.

However, it may be a very long time before the origins of some of these diseases are discovered; and even when they are, there may be difficulties – behavioural, technical, economic – in achieving control. It is therefore essential to have further knowledge of disease processes from clinical and laboratory research to provide treatment of established disorders, and in some cases, no doubt, produce a complete solution.

INVESTIGATION OF DISEASE MECHANISMS

Although I believe that the solution of most disease problems will come in the future, as in the past, from control of disease origins, I hope I have left no doubt about my recognition of the continued importance of research aimed at increasing our understanding of disease mechanisms. At the risk that it will be considered an act of supererogation, I will summarize the grounds for this view.

1. It is unthinkable that man, who is keenly interested in the nature of the world in which he lives and the contents of the space beyond it, should not have an equal or greater interest in his own body and the diseases which affect it.

2. Whatever doubts one may have about the possibility of eliminating many diseases through knowledge of their mechanisms in the foreseeable future, in the light of past experience of the unpredictability of scientific progress it would be foolish to set limits on what may one day be possible.

3. There is one class of medical problems, and that arguably the most difficult (referred to above as 'relatively intractable'), in which only a mechanistic approach is likely to succeed.

4. The control of diseases which are in principle preventable may be delayed, in some cases indefinitely, for a number of reasons: because the influences are largely unknown (as is the case at this time in breast cancer and multiple sclerosis); because they are multiple, and hence difficult to dissociate (as in coronary artery disease); because they are costly to eliminate (as in many accidents and occupational hazards); because their control involves changes in behaviour which people are reluctant to accept (as in cancer of the lung and cirrhosis of the liver); because they

are technically complex (as in malaria and schistosomiasis). So long as the deleterious influences are not eliminated there will be a need for continued treatment of diseases and disabilities which are in principle avoidable. Indeed, some of the greatest successes of clinical medicine, based on a knowledge of disease mechanisms, are from treatment of conditions such as accidents which, ideally, should not occur.

13

Dream, Mirage or Nemesis?

In Dostoevsky's novel *The Possessed* there is a hilarious chapter which describes a meeting of provincial liberals who have assembled to hear a message from two prominent radicals. Unfortunately the great men seem less interested in revolution than in brandy and cards, and the conversation becomes trivial, heated, confused, irrelevant to the great issues they have come to hear discussed. Finally the host despairingly begs someone to make a statement, and they proceed to vote on the question whether they are a meeting in some formal sense, or merely a group of friends who have met to celebrate a name-day.

In medicine also there is confusion but, by contrast, no lack of statements; indeed there is a surfeit of them. Unfortunately for the earnest seeker after truth they are by no means consistent and some are frankly contradictory. (One is reminded of the opening paragraph of *A Tale of Two Cities*: 'It was the best of times, it was the worst of times . . .'). So we are told on the one hand that medical science has already achieved miracles and that if we will only provide the resources and have a little patience it will shortly solve all our problems, and on the other that an exact evaluation of twentieth-century medicine would do much to restore nineteenth-century faith in prayer. It is said that many countries already enjoy a high standard of health which will soon be raised further, and, on the contrary, that with changing conditions of life disease problems must also be expected to change and the goal of improved health is largely illusory. The doctor is described as a man of principle devoted to the advancement of science and the welfare of his patients, and as a charlatan who can be counted on to look after nothing but his own interests.

Some of the scepticism is perhaps no more than good-natured banter of the kind to which the professions seem particularly exposed; certainly no worse than things that are said about clergymen and a good deal kinder than many reflections on the work of lawyers. But whatever the motivation in the past there is undoubtedly a new note of severity in contempory criticism; the critics, or at least some of them, mean what they say. Here, for example, are the observations of Nancy Mitford on the work of doctors at the time of Louis XIV and today.

The fashionable doctors . . . stood as they do now, in admiration of their own science. As now, they talked as if illness and death were mastered. Molière has presented that sort of doctor once and for all; a consultation of big-wigs is ever a scene from one of his plays. The learned, magic, meaningless words, the grave looks at each other, the artful hesitation between one worthless formula and another—all are there. In those days, terrifying in black robes and bonnets they bled the patient; now terrifying in white robes and masks they pump blood into him. The result is the same; the strong live; the weak, after much suffering and expense, both of spirit and money, die.[1]

Such criticisms should be taken seriously, and for a number of reasons. In the first place, there is a good deal of truth in the allegations. Doctors have always tended to overestimate the effectiveness of their intervention and to underestimate the risks, whether removing large quantities of blood, under mistaken notions of the blood volume, in the treatment of yellow fever in the eighteenth century, or exposing patients to dangerous levels of radiation, of whose effects they were unaware, when screening for breast cancer in the twentieth. There was and is still a good deal of unjustified complacency about the extent of understanding of disease and of ability to control it, for example, in the assumptions that malaria and schistosomiasis will soon be eradicated or that there is little more to fear from airborne infections. And patients have been and continue to be exposed to pain and injury from misguided attempts to do them good. Suffering is only marginally more tolerable when inflicted with the best intentions, and the death of Charles II under treatment by his doctors was much more cruel than that of his father at the hands of his executioner. Indeed the history of treatment of illness in the aristocracy,[2] who were able to obtain the 'best' medical care, suggests that Francis Galton was generous in his conclusion that there is a considerable difference between a good doctor and a bad one, but hardly any difference between a good doctor and none at all.

A second reason for reappraisal of the role of doctors is the more independent line now taken by other health professionals. In some respects this is less a result of a fresh assessment of the needs of patients

1. Mitford, N., *The Sun King* (London: Sphere Books Ltd, 1969), p. 141.
2. Excellently recorded for the French Court in the Memoirs of Saint-Simon.

than an expression of the spirit of our times, when notions of equality and freedom are applied in all circumstances, even to the relation between parents and children. But it is also true that nurses, social workers, hygienists, and others have come to believe that they can often function just as effectively without the advice, and much more happily without the supervision of the doctor.

There is also a change in public attitudes to medicine, less evident in Britain than in the United States. In that country the image of the doctor as a devoted healer has been shaken by the resistance of professional organizations to the introduction of publicly financed and administered health services, and by the unwillingness of doctors to practise in areas which they find unattractive: even, in some cases, where patients are able to meet the costs of private medical care. To many people doctors seem less concerned about the welfare of patients than about their own convenience and standard of living. In such circumstances insistence on the delicacy of the doctor–patient relationship by the physician seems an anomaly, equivalent to the suggestion that the privacy of the confessional is intended to protect, not the sinner but the priest.

As noted in an earlier chapter, these reactions to the doctor's position have been muted to some extent by the belief that his role is critical for the health of patients. When it becomes generally known, as surely it will, that the determinants of health are largely outside the medical care system, the questions are likely to become even more insistent. If we are neither cured when we are ill nor well cared for when we are disabled, what is the role of medicine in which so much has been invested, in hope and resources?

I have put the question in the provocative form in which it may be asked, indeed in which it has already been asked by some who have lost faith in the work of doctors. But if the question is overstated so too are likely to be the answers. From the belief that medicine can do everything, opinion is in danger of swinging to the equally untenable conclusion that it can do little or nothing. It is therefore important for the public as well as for the profession itself, that the medical role should be reconsidered, fairly and objectively, taking account of both its achievements in the past and its probable contributions in the foreseeable future.

Before examining the medical role I shall refer to four books which raise many of the important issues. They are *The Lives of a Cell*,[3]

3. Thomas, L., *The Lives of a Cell* (Toronto, New York, London: Bantam Books Inc., 1975).

Genes, Dreams and Realities,[4] *The Mirage of Health,*[5] and *Medical Nemesis.*[6]

DREAM

Perhaps the most common opinion is that medicine has already solved many disease problems, and if it is not yet in sight of a solution of all that remain, it is unquestionably on the right lines. There is also the modified view that the dream has faded, that formerly there were great achievements, but what remains is much less impressive, the 'degenerate remnant of something immense in the past'.[7] On the first interpretation there is little need for a change of direction, but on the second a reappraisal of the medical role is clearly required.

The more cheerful conclusion was expressed with due caution by Thomas in terms which would probably be acceptable to most medical scientists. He suggested that 'the great contemporary achievement of modern medicine is the technology for controlling and preventing bacterial infection', and he cited as examples 'immunisation against diphtheria, pertussis (and the childhood virus diseases) and the contemporary use of antibiotics and chemotherapy for bacterial infections' such as syphilis and tuberculosis. Thomas recognized the limitations of medical measures: 'For all the new knowledge, we still have formidable diseases, still unsolved, lacking satisfactory explanation, lacking satisfactory treatment'; and 'In real life, the biomedical sciences have not yet reached the stage of any kind of general applicability to disease mechanisms.' Significantly, he saw a parallel with the physical sciences of the early twentieth century, 'booming along into new territory, but without an equivalent for the engineering of the time'. However, he doubted whether the further development of an applied science in medicine can be hurried, and suggested that 'the greatest part of the important biomedical research waiting to be done is in the class of basic science'.[8]

The grounds for one's reservations about this interpretation were

4. Burnet, Sir Macfarlane, *Genes, Dreams and Realities* (Aylesbury, Bucks: Medical and Technical Publishing Co. Ltd, 1971).

5. Dubos, R., *The Mirage of Health* (London: George Allen and Unwin Ltd, 1960).

6. Illich, I., *Medical Nemesis* (London: Calder and Boyars Ltd, 1975).

7. Auden, W. H., *Poems* (London: Faber and Faber Ltd, 1934), p. 64. (Auden's version of Chekhov's 'the shrinking remnant of something which was once enormous'.)

8. Thomas, L., *The Lives of a Cell.*

discussed in previous chapters and need not be repeated at length. But briefly, with the possible exception of diphtheria, mortality from the common infections (tuberculosis, pneumonia, scarlet fever, measles, pertussis, etc.) had declined to quite a low level before effective immunization and chemotherapy became available. The largest contribution of biomedical science was the extension of hygienic measures made possible by understanding of disease and identification of micro-organisms. Control of the infections resulted mainly from modification of the conditions under which they occurred, and there are theoretical as well as historical reasons for believing that the same approach is required for an attack on many of the disease problems that remain.

Very different views were expressed by a distinguished micro-biologist in *Genes, Dreams and Realities*. Burnet suggested 'that future historians may speak of an age of scientific discovery that started with Galileo in 1586 and ended something less than four hundred years later'. He implied that laboratory research made a large contribution in the past, but cannot be expected to do so in future, when the most important challenges will be the so-called 'intrinsic' types of disease and disability (cancer, old-age, and auto-immune disease), diseases of civilization (lung cancer, road accidents, alcoholism, drug addiction, etc.), and the general problems of society which impinge on health: limitation of population growth, disarmament, and control of the environment. In solving such problems laboratory medicine has little to offer, and pride of place in biology is now held by the observational sciences, ecology and ethology, 'because of their rather direct bearing on contempory human problems'.[9]

Broadly, Burnet's views seem closer to those of Thomas in respect of the past and to those expressed in this book in respect of the future. Although he recognized that 'The accelerating increase of human populations since the eighteenth century has depended mainly on two factors, an increase in the amount of food available and the development, incidentally or deliberately, of ways of diminishing infectious disease', he suggested that specific measures of prevention (DDT and other potent insecticides), immunization, and treatment 'have changed a steady population increase into an explosion'. While this may be true (particularly of DDT and insecticides) in developing countries today, it is not accurate for the developed countries in the past three centuries, when the decline of mortality and growth of population were essentially

9. Burnet, Sir Macfarlane, *Genes, Dreams and Realities*.

independent of specific measures. The interpretation, therefore, somewhat overstates the contribution of laboratory medicine in the past; it may also underestimate its value in the future: for example, it is by no means unlikely that amniocentesis and related measures discovered mainly by laboratory research will make it possible to recognize and eliminate many serious abnormalities before birth. But the general conclusions, that many diseases and disabilities determined at fertilization will remain intractable, and that most abnormalities attributable to conditions of life will be controlled by modification of those conditions rather than through laboratory investigation, seem unexceptionable. However, an epidemiologist is unlikely to be persuaded that the interest and the usefulness of the tasks confronting the research worker no longer coincide.

MIRAGE

One of the most interesting ideas related to the medical role is the notion that the goal of improved health is to some extent illusory, a mirage which inspires and attracts but will continue to elude us, however diligently we seek it. This concept was outlined by Dubos in *The Mirage of Health*,[10] and stated explicitly in a later book:

It is a dangerous error to believe that disease and suffering can be wiped out altogether by raising still further the standards of living, increasing our mastery of the environment, and developing new therapeutic procedures. The less pleasant reality is that, since the world is ever changing, each period and each type of civilisation will continue to have its burden of diseases created by the unavoidable failure of biological and social adaptation to counter new environmental threats.[11]

This interpretation seems consistent with man's history until the last three centuries. During most of his existence he lived as a nomad, dependent on fortuitous food sources and, like other animals in their natural habitats, subject to rigorous natural selection which kept disease at a low frequency. With small populations at low densities infectious diseases as we have known them in the historical period were not a serious problem, and illness and early death were determined by the primitive conditions of life: food shortage, homicide, accidents, and predation.

10. Dubos, R., *The Mirage of Health.*
11. Dubos, R., *Man, Medicine, and Environment* (London: Pall Mall Press, 1968), p. 85.

The first Agricultural Revolution ten thousand years ago led to profound changes. A settled way of life and domestication of plants and animals increased food supplies and resulted in population growth. The aggregation of large populations created the conditions needed for the propagation and transmission of micro-organisms, particularly those that were air-, water-, and food-borne. However, with unrestricted growth of population food supplies became again marginal, so that lack of food was once more an important source of ill-health. But there was this difference from the earlier period, that infectious diseases had become the predominant cause of sickness and death.

To this point, roughly to 1700, experience seems entirely consistent with the view that as conditions of life change we move from one set of health problems to another: 'We owe God a death. He that dies this year is quit for the next.'[12] But is the interpretation equally valid when applied to the last three centuries, and what is even more important: does it suggest that there are strict limits to the health goals that can be reached in future?

Perhaps the first point which should be made is that it is a very restricted view of life which can be obtained by inspection of death certificates. Everyone must die, but it makes a great difference whether the deaths are in early, middle, or late life. The changes since 1700 resulted in a large increase in expectation of life, reflected in a transfer of deaths from early to late life. The transformation of causes of sickness and death during the past three centuries cannot therefore be described accurately as the exchange of one set of health problems for another.

In developing countries today the predominant infectious diseases can also be dealt with by measures which do not of themselves create health problems of another kind. However, it is a short step from sufficient food to a surfeit, and in the developed world a new set of problems has appeared, essentially those associated with the changes of behaviour which are possible in an affluent society. Are these problems which appear after the decline of the infections likely to be solved without creating new ones?

The residual problems vary greatly in their character. Those determined at fertilization or by prenatal influences have been little affected by recent changes, and are probably neither more nor less tractable than they were before. Those due to lack of food or environmental hazards can be resolved by an extension of measures which have been successful

12. *Henry IV, Part II.*

hitherto, although this will require strict control of new risks, particularly those associated with industrial processes and medical procedures. The possibility that one group of health problems has been exchanged for another arises most seriously in relation to the diseases of affluence. They appear to be due largely to a departure from conditions of life under which man evolved, and the question is whether a return to those conditions in order to prevent them is feasible.

In some cases there is no obvious reason why it should not be. Both health and quality of life are improved by taking exercise, avoiding tobacco and other drugs, and limiting consumption of alcohol and food. As these are now the main determinants of health it is hard to believe that society will not wish to create conditions under which such practices are encouraged. In many ways the problems are epitomized by smoking, where the serious damage to health of large numbers of people has to be weighed against the commercial and other interests which will suffer if smoking is reduced and finally stopped.

A problem which differs only in degree is that of traffic accidents. It is unlikely that society will accept elimination of motor vehicles, although their limitation and stricter control will be inevitable, not only for health reasons. What does seem unacceptable is a high level of accidents due to drinking and driving, and stringent measures have already been introduced, for example in Sweden.

A class of health problems for which it is perhaps most difficult to see a possible solution are those related to changes in reproductive behaviour. The infections due to promiscuity can conceivably be controlled by preventive measures or treatment; but it is possible that the profound changes in reproduction associated with the fall of the birth-rate since the nineteenth century have contributed to the prevalence of breast cancer and other diseases of the reproductive system. If so, these abnormalities truly represent the problem to which Dubos referred, the appearance of new diseases as a consequence of the conditions which led to the decline of the old ones. Society may very well return to some of our ancesttral practices, for example by increasing exercise, reducing fat consumption, and replacing refined flour by whole meal. It would find it much more difficult to accept early and frequent pregnancies, should it be shown that these are the changes needed to reduce the frequency of cancer of the breast.

While it is true that disease and suffering cannot be wiped out, particularly those forms determined at fertilization or by prenatal influences, experience of the past three centuries shows that it is possible to achieve an enormous improvement in health by modification of post-natal influences. Of the three which have been most effective, increased food supplies, control of hazards, and limitation of numbers, only the last may be associated with a new set of disease problems, brought about by the change in reproductive practice. However, the wealth which led to the improvement of nutrition and hygiene has made it possible to depart radically from the conditions under which man evolved, by over-eating, under–exercising, smoking, and the like. Whether future progress in health will be restricted by these changes will depend on whether men are prepared to modify their life styles and follow the principles by which some dissenting minorities have lived for centuries. Perhaps the ideal to which we should aspire is that of the Quaker of moderate but firm convictions, who believes that it is permissible, even desirable to have wealth so long as it is not abused. Shaw touched on the same point in the Preface to *Man and Superman* when he wrote: 'Do not waste your time on Social Questions. What is the matter with the poor is Poverty. What is the matter with the rich is Uselessness.' It has taken hundreds of thousands of years to remove the ill-health associated with poverty, and we should not be surprised if it takes a little time to remove that which is associated with wealth. But there is no reason for despondency on the grounds that we have merely exchanged one set of health problems for another.

NEMESIS

A third suggestion to be considered is that the role of medicine is essentially sinister. It should not surprise us, for it has been made before; but in terms so benign that the offence of what was said was quite removed by the manner of saying it. People, including medical people, were more amused than provoked when Shaw described the medical service as a murderous absurdity, and referred to the physician as, among other things, a credulous imposter, petulent scientific coxcomb, and parasite on disease. In Illich's *Medical Nemesis* the conclusions are much the same but the tone is different; with passion and without humour he described the medical role as a threat, to society as well as patients, that can only be removed by a public unfrocking of the offending practitioners.[13]

The grounds for this proposal are said to be threefold: medicine does more harm than good; it breeds demands for its services and supports

13. Illich, I., *Medical Nemesis*.

features of society which generate ill-health; most seriously, it diminishes the capacity of the individual to deal with his own health problems and to face suffering and death. Let us consider them in turn.

1. The assertion that 'a professional and physician-based health care system . . . must produce clinical damages which outweigh its practical benefits' is rather like a statement that there is more evil than good in the world. There may be; but there is no means of proving or disproving it, and in both the medical and the celestial balance sheets the decision must turn on definitions and value judgements. My own impression, for what it is worth, is that if the term medicine is taken to include the whole enterprise – nutritional, hygienic, and behavioural as well as therapeutic – there is little doubt that the balance is strongly in medicine's favour. If it is restricted to clinical services, the answer varies from place to place and from physician to physician. Certainly there are countries where one would not like to be ill, and there are doctors in all countries by whom one would prefer not to be treated. But there are others to whom one would go unhesitatingly with a disease problem, confident that the advice would be sound and the treatment, if indicated, beneficial and never harmful. The conclusion that clinical damages *must* outweigh the benefits is mistaken, and if they sometimes do the answer is to make the services better rather than to blow them up. It is perhaps worth noting that Illich was misinformed about the value of some of the procedures to which he refers: the decline of pneumonia is not attributable mainly to sulphonamides and antibiotics; although treatment of typhoid is effective the disease cannot be said to be cured quite easily; vaccines have contributed little to the decline of deaths from whooping cough and measles; the effect of replacement therapy on diabetes is not only in the short run; the value of vaginal smears in intervention for cervical cancer has not been proved; and the effectiveness of drug treatment of high blood pressure is not restricted to patients with malignant hypertension. There are some advantages in having medical experience when assessing medical procedures.

2. It is well recognized that the demand for clinical services increases with their availability; just as some children can occupy the attention of as many adults as are prepared to wait on them, some patients appear to require the services of as many doctors as can be persuaded to see them. But the conclusion that on this account physician services as we know them should cease, is rather like the suggestion that because some people overeat there should be no more baking of bread. Of course there is a problem of restricting demand for a wide range of consumer

services, but it will not be solved simply by bringing them to an end.

It is more difficult to come to grips with the second point under the same heading: that health policies reinforce an industrial organization which generates ill-health. Like another passionate critic of health services (Enoch Powell[14]), Illich gives an impression of lucidity while sometimes leaving one in doubt about the precise meaning of what he is saying. It is not obvious that medical intervention contributes to two of the main determinants of ill-health – lack of food and environmental hazards; and belief in the value of treatment probably has little effect on the predominant behavioural influences – for example, the mistaken idea that doctors can cure cancer of the lung and chronic bronchitis is not in the mind of the adolescent when he begins smoking. Illich refers in the same context to a different point: the survival of increasing numbers of defectives who require institutional care. Only a very small part of this problem is attributable to misguided medical intervention, such as surgical treatment of children seriously handicapped by spina bifida; the large majority of mentally retarded people now survive, not because of specific medical measures, but because society is unwilling to withhold from them the basic necessities of life. For many of us the solution of the problem of the congenitally handicapped, if and when there is one, lies not in denial of humane care, but in avoidance of their conception or birth.

3. Illich seems to attach most importance to his third point: that medical services reduce the capacity of the individual to care for himself and to face suffering and death. He appears to believe that medical procedures fall broadly into two classes: those that are cheap, effective, and simple, so that the patient could apply them himself; and those that are expensive, complicated, and useless, so that little would be lost if they were abandoned. In this reading there would be only occasional need for 'specialized healers', although presumably they would have to advise patients from time to time whether their services were necessary: like the doctor in Mary Baker Eddy's biography, called to see a sick Christian Scientist who was no better after several hours of intensive prayer, and told that he was not to do anything, but merely to ascertain what should be prayed for.

There are many things people should do for their health but they are not those that Illich has chiefly in mind. I believe they should recognize that they are healthy and live in such a way that they remain so; he

14. A former Minister of Health in Britain.

emphasizes their frailty, and would like them to take over their treatment and, when this fails, bear with their suffering.

The notion that the application of effective treatment is usually simple is mistaken. Isoniazid, one of the most valuable therapeutic agents, is easily administered; but it is necessary first to be sure that the patient has tuberculosis and that is not a simple matter. Antibiotics are commonly misused by doctors in treatment of respiratory diseases; they are even more likely to be abused by the public who can hardly be expected to distinguish clearly between viral and bacterial infections. Some of the most useful procedures, such as treatment of accidents, dental conditions, and unpredictable obstetric emergencies, require both specialized equipment and professional skill. But more generally, the gross abuse of drugs already available to the public gives no ground for confidence that if medical control (by no means wholly effective) were withdrawn all would be well; indeed it is probable that the harm which results from self-administered sedatives, analgesics, tranquillizers, etc., not to mention tobacco, alcohol, and opiates is already far greater than that caused by medical intervention.

The most complex matter is the attitude to pain and suffering which is not only, or mainly, a health-related question. The ideas about suffering are very ancient: Epicurus maintained that a man could be happy on the rack and wrote on the day of his death: 'On this truly happy day of my life, as I am on the point of death, I write this to you. The diseases of my bladder and stomach are pursuing their course, lacking nothing of their usual severity: but against all this is the joy in my heart at the recollection of my conversations with you.' The Stoics taught endurance rather than hope; cruelty and injustice should not be resented since they provide excellent opportunities for the practice of virtue, and medical men are unnecessary because illness is not an evil. 'I must die. But must I die groaning?' Epictetus asked, and he held that happiness resulted from 'the sense that your affairs depend on no one'. Related ideas are to be found in St Augustine and Tolstoy, both of whom were obsessed by a sense of sin, original and self-engendered, which could be expurgated only by suffering. The significance of misery was central to Pascal's thought: 'La connaissance de Dieu sans celle de notre misère fait l'orgueil; la connaissance de notre misère sans celle de Jésus-Christ fait le désespoir.' Kierkegaard wrote with satisfaction: 'The human race has in the course of generations become even more insignificant', and he and others have implied that the world would be the poorer if pain and suffering were eliminated.

There are at least three ideas interwoven in these reflections: pain and misery are inescapable (Pascal); they are rewarding (St Augustine and Tolstoy); and one should prepare to face them (Epicurus and Epictetus). If these views are accepted there is obviously little to be said for employing professional healers whose task is to relieve distress.

When Pascal wrote of 'notre misère' he referred to mental as well as physical suffering; in the present context it will be sufficiently ambitious to restrict attention to the latter. The idea that pain and suffering are inevitable is I think mistaken: it was probably true, or very nearly so, for most of man's life on earth; but with the provision of sufficient food and control of hazards in the past few centuries, many people have completed their lives without severe or prolonged physical discomfort. It is also true that medicine can contribute largely to the relief of suffering when it occurs, and even saints and reformed sinners would accept anaesthesia for removal of an impacted third molar, and surgical intervention for treatment of a perforated peptic ulcer or obstructed labour.

The conclusion that physical suffering is not inevitable and can often be relieved when it occurs does not of course meet the objection that pain is rewarding and should be accepted, even sought rather than resisted. Such ideas usually come from people of exceptional sensitivity and imagination who should be careful about prescribing for others who are less gifted or less afflicted than themselves. A man may say paradoxically: I find life a misery yet dread the prospect of death; I can come to terms with existence only if I resign myself to pain and suffering. But except on religious grounds, which can be accepted or rejected he should not pass the same harsh sentence on other people (I suspect the large majority) who do not share his anguish, and find severe and prolonged suffering, like severe and prolonged poverty, degrading rather than elevating. Moreover response to distress is not unrelated to the background and condition of the individual who bears it. It is one thing to give up wealth, like Francis of Assisi, and quite another never to have had it. After a period of debauchery, repentance at Yasnaya Polyana must have been more refreshing for its master than for one of his servants, and the down-and-outness of an Old Etonian who subsequently put his experience into a book[15] was very different from that of a peasant who fled from rural poverty in East Bengal to urban squalor on the streets of Calcutta. It would be unfortunate if the prescription for bearing the ills of the flesh were to be written by those who bear

15. Orwell, G., *Down and Out in Paris and London* (London: Secker and Warburg, 1949).

mainly the ills of the mind, for there are many more suffering peasants than there are Tolstoys and Orwells.

Accommodation to life's minor trials is another matter. An obstetrician at the hospital where I trained as a medical student used to tell of a Spanish town that went into mourning when the blinds were drawn at the great house to indicate that its mistress was having her period. There is something to be said for the view that people should not thrust their problems unreasonably on others, for although Freud's teaching is appropriate to great suffering, the advice of Moody and Sankey – 'Go bury thy sorrow, the world hath its share' – is more in keeping with the requirements of everyday life.

14

Medicine as an Institution

Having touched on various ideas related to the medical role, I must now try to bring them together in a more coherent form. Before doing so, however, it will be desirable to remove some possible sources of misunderstanding.

First, the aim of health services. We know from personal experience that the feeling of well-being, sometimes referred to as positive health, is something more than the absence of recognizable disease and disability, and it is tempting to define objectives, as the World Health Organization has defined them, in terms which recognize this.[1] However, there are at least two objections to so broad a definition: one, that positive health cannot be measured accurately, so that success or failure in achieving it can only be judged subjectively; the other, that since many influences, personal, religious, educational, and economic as well as medical, contribute to a state of well-being, the concept goes far beyond the responsibilities of health services. I shall therefore define the aim more modestly as the prevention of sickness and premature death and the care of the sick and disabled. In these terms the task of medicine is not to create happiness, but so far as possible to remove a major source of unhappiness, that which results from illness and early death.

By this definition, medicine is concerned both with improving the quality of life and with extending its duration, in so far as these aims can be achieved by preventing or treating disease. (This is quite different from attempting to increase the normal life span.) However, some people have suggested that only the first aim is realistic. In an interesting review of prospects for clinical pharmacology, Modell concluded:

It should be the primary function of clinical pharmacology in the last quarter of this century to secure the achievements in drug therapy of the preceding half

1. In the constitution of the World Health Organization health was defined as a 'state of complete physical, mental and social well-being and not merely the absence of disease or infirmity'.

century. ... We must also make life more tolerable. Drugs for the relief of symptoms rather than etiology is a goal truly worthy of intensive study and originally the only realistic goal of medicine. ... I think that these goals have a better chance of success in the future than attempts to reduce the death-rate further or lengthen the lifespan.[2]

These views are based on recognition that the therapeutic advances of the last few decades have had little effect on death rates, and that in developed countries we are approaching the 'normal' lifespan which medicine cannot be expected to extend. One can accept both conclusions without agreeing that cure is no longer a realistic aim. The patient with a life threatening illness – malignant hypertension, multiple sclerosis, leukaemia, nephritis etc. – wishes above all to be restored to a life of normal duration, and this is a goal which deserves to be rated at least equally with improvements in quality of life. This conclusion is not invalidated because extension of life in such diseases could not be expected to have much effect on national death rates from all causes, or on life expectancy at birth, since the numbers of people affected by the diseases is small in relation to the total population, and many illnesses occur in late life when the possible addition of years is limited. Success in prolonging life from a specific disease should be assessed in relation to those affected, rather than to the general population.

At the outset I should like to sidestep the trade union disputes which arise over the role of the doctor in relation to other health workers. These roles are changing, and at some future time the respective trainings and responsibilities of the physician and nurse in primary care, and of the physician and social worker in care of the subnormal, may be quite different from those which exist today. When commenting on the medical role I am therefore referring to the work done by doctors and others concerned with 'prevention of sickness and premature death and care of the sick and disabled', and I am not specifying or implying any unique role for the physician. My concern is with the work to be done rather than with who should do it.

Finally, it is important to remove a common source of misunderstanding, by distinguishing clearly between clinical practice on the one hand and the larger responsibilities of medicine as an institution on the other.

For many people this distinction scarcely exists. Medicine is the profession of doctors, and doctors are thought to be concerned essentially

2. Modell, W., 'Clinical Pharmacology: a retrospective view of its future', *Triangle*, **16** (1977), p. 123.

with the diagnosis and treatment of disease in individual patients. Having this role, they cannot be held responsible for health maintenance in well people, or for the work of non-personal services in the community at large. It is not a denial of the importance of these services to recognize that they are incompatible with clinical practice, and hence, it is concluded, they fall outside medicine's responsibilities.

This interpretation results from equating medicine as an institution with clinical practice. Of course the doctor who treats sick people cannot be expected to deal with national food policies, changes in the environment and public attempts to modify behaviour, although an understanding of these influences on health seems at least as relevant to his work as knowledge of the chemistry of the drugs he uses. But there are serious objections to limiting the institutional role of medicine in the same way. Medicine would no longer be concerned comprehensively with health matters, and there would be a particularly regrettable division between professions dealing with the prevention and treatment of disease. Education and training of health workers of different types would become even more widely separated than at the present time, and medical research would be increasingly polarized towards investigation of disease mechanisms, with serious risk of neglect of disease origins. It is indeed one of the most unfortunate features of the contemporary professional organizations (colleges, faculties, associations, societies) that they represent sectional interests and collectively provide no forum for consideration of the larger issues which should be the concern of medicine as an institution.

For these and other reasons the role of medicine as an institution should be considered to cover prevention as well as treatment of disease, and to include concern with non-personal as well as personal services. I suggest that it should be interpreted as follows: To assist us to come safely into the world and comfortably out of it, and during life to protect the well and care for the sick and disabled.

SAFELY INTO THE WORLD

Since I shall certainly be told that we can come into the world (and out of it) without medical assistance, I have taken care to suggest for medicine only a supplementary role. But under it I am referring to much more than the act of delivery itself: to prevention of the birth of the seriously abnormal, and to limitation of the number of births, as well as the safeguarding of normal pregnancy and labour.

I do not think medicine has anything to contribute in relation to such questionable and technically remote objectives as selection of parents in order to improve the human race. But it is reasonable to identify parents whose likelihood of having a seriously abnormal birth can be specified – for example to tell those who have had a child with a malformation of the heart or central nervous system that the risk of malformation in a later birth is increased above the average risk, but is still relatively low. It would be even better if it were possible to specify the risk of congenital abnormalities for parents who have not previously had an abnormal child; but since the common ones are probably determined by intra-uterine conditions, this is not at present a very promising objective.

Identification of deleterious influences during pregnancy is equally important, and perhaps equally difficult. Nevertheless it is possible that other agents such as thalidomide and rubella will be discovered, and if they are external to the uterus they may be easily removed. Influences arising within the uterus are much more difficult to recognize and control.

On the basis of present knowledge, or of any probable extension of it, neither of these approaches – identification of parents likely to have abnormal births or of deleterious influences during pregnancy which can be removed – offers much prospect of control of most serious congenital conditions. It is therefore important to seek means of recognizing the abnormal foetus in early pregnancy when it can be aborted.

Doctors have no more and no less right than other people to define the limits of population growth, but the limits having been defined they have a role in the prevention of conception and termination of pregnancy, unless, as Illich suggests, abortion is to be managed on a do-it-yourself basis.[3] In making this proposal he underestimates the technical difficulties, particularly the risk of infection and of later complications.

Clear thinking is needed about the contribution of medicine to the conduct of normal pregnancy and labour. It is quite true that the large majority of people have come into the world without professional assistance, but the mortality of mothers and children was very high until the present century. It is also true that mortality can be reduced dramatically by relatively simple measures, particularly in literate populations which enjoy a high standard of living. In most developed countries maternal mortality is now very low and perinatal and infant mortality are both about 20 (per 1,000). But the difference between low

3. Illich, I., *Medical Nemesis*.

rates and the lowest rates is determined by the handling of occasional unforeseen emergencies which require facilities and skill of the kind available in hospitals. A society which wishes to get the best results will therefore need to provide simple care for all pregnancies with more sophisticated measures in reserve for the unpredictable complications.

PROTECTION OF THE WELL

The conclusion which I hope emerges from the preceding chapters is that the improvement in health hitherto has been due predominantly to protection of people born free of congenital disabilities, and that it is to the same approach that we must look mainly for the solution of the residual problems of the common diseases. Most of those who are born well will remain well, apart from minor morbidity, at least until late life, if they have enough to eat, if they are not exposed to serious hazards, and if they do not injure themselves by unwise behaviour, particularly by departing radically from the conditions under which man evolved.

What part has medicine to play in achieving these objectives? First, since doctors are concerned more comprehensively with human health than any other professional group, they should make it their business to know and to make known, the relative importance of the major influences. Second, the medical contribution in the fields of nutrition and environmental health, where the measures are essentially non-personal, should be in the hands of specialists, who need to be attracted to these subjects as undergraduates and trained in them as graduates. The responsibility which falls on doctors who provide personal care is that of influencing their patients' behaviour in relation to their health. Having regard for the determinants of health a doctor can say to himself quite accurately: In pursuit of the major objectives of preventing sickness and premature death, I can often do more for my patients, particularly young patients, by persuading them to modify their habits than by any treatment that can be offered. The scope for this approach will be even greater when more is known about the common diseases, particularly in the field of mental health where investigation of the major influences has scarcely begun.

CARE OF THE SICK AND DISABLED

Under this heading I include all aspects of care: investigation and treatment of acute illness as well as rehabilitation and prolonged care.

Until the present time the emphasis in medicine has been on only a part of this task, on the kind of work done in acute hospitals: investigation of disease, treatment of acute illness or of acute phases of chronic illness, and treatment of some non-acute conditions (such as hernias, piles, and varicose veins).

At first sight it is not easy to see what determines these interests and excludes others; for example, there is less concern with acute illness in the severly handicapped (the congenitally malformed, the mentally ill, the subnormal, and the very old). Since the eighteenth century the administrations and staffs of general hospitals would have said that they took patients who could make the best use of their resources; but this is not a convincing explanation, since some are admitted who derive little or no benefit, while others are excluded who could be helped. I suggest that there are at least three determinants of the admissions policies of acute hospitals which both reflect and influence the interests of their staffs: they prefer patients who are acutely ill, who are not permanently handicapped, and who provide scope for the current range of investigative and therapeutic procedures. At the present time, with the enormous growth of technology the last is possibly the main determinant; even mongols are occasionally admitted now that they have been shown to have interesting chromosomes.

It is, I believe, a fair criticism of the selective medical interests, that they lead to the neglect of some patients, indeed of the majority, and to concern with only a limited part of the needs of those who are helped. But the omissions had this justification, that the work in the acute phase of an illness was thought to be critical and largely responsible for the modern improvement in health.

This assumption was mistaken. The treatment of established disease, although important for patients, does not usually restore them to a life of normal duration and quality; and the modern improvement in health was due to the prevention of disease rather than to treatment after it occurred.

The conclusion to be drawn is that the achievements of the acute hospital do not justify the relative neglect of the majority of hospital patients who are not admitted. Three things are needed: (*a*) a critical appraisal of the effectiveness and efficiency of procedures already in use or to be brought into use; (*b*) recognition that investigation and treatment of the acute episode does not usually change the underlying condition, and that the patient needs advice and care throughout his illness; (*c*) a reshaping of services which removes the arbitrary divisions between the patients in acute, mental, chronic, and mental subnormality hospitals.

I have discussed the approach to effectiveness and efficiency in Chapter 10. On the second point, treatment of patients, in these days usually elderly patients, in acute episodes of heart disease, cancer, pneumonia, etc., is not a sufficient basis for the main work of a hospital, still less for a concept of the essence of the medical task. This service is vital to the patients concerned, but it often fails to meet their requirements in the later stages of the illness, or in the months and years which follow when they are no longer in the acute phase. I have written elsewhere at length on the third point, about the origins and consequences of the separation of acute from mental and other hospitals.[4] In the present context all that need be added is that the differences in standards have no justification in the different contributions the hospitals are making to the care of the sick and disabled.

COMFORTABLY OUT OF THE WORLD

I refer here not only to terminal care in the period immediately before death, but also to the assistance of patients who may be disabled for months or years before their final illness. Although elderly patients with prolonged incapacity are seen frequently in general practice and in hospital, many people complete their lives without serious handicap from chronic disease or disability.[5]

The health and related social services need to make much better provision for chronic and terminal care. Both have been relatively neglected, partly because the work is unattractive to many doctors, but also because it is considered less important than investigation and treatment of acute illness. The elderly patient and his relatives cannot be expected to see it in this way. The diagnosis of untreatable cancer (for example) is necessary, but meets only a small fragment of the patient's needs in the months or years which follow. And although most people end their lives without a prolonged period of incapacity, many welcome medical attention in their last illness. Their relatives almost invariably do.

Some centres are concerned with terminal care, and a few devote

4. McKeown, T., *Medicine in Modern Society* (London: George Allen and Unwin Ltd, 1965).

5. Sheldon, J. H., *The Social Medicine of Old Age* (London: Oxford University Press, 1948).

themselves entirely to patients who face extreme physical and mental distress in their last illness. In effect they are saying: Give us the worst that can happen, and we will show that when professional skill is combined with humane care, the last days of life can be made tolerable, even cheerful, for the most afflicted people. Their work is beyond praise; but it should be taken as an example rather than a model, for the size and character of the problem is such that it cannot be divorced from the rest of medical care. Doctors need to regard prolonged and terminal care as an important and rewarding part of their task which should not be transferred to other people or to special institutions. For the patient and relatives the medical contribution at the end of life is as significant as attempts made at an earlier stage to protect or prolong it.

CONCLUSIONS

In the broadest terms, the medical role is in three areas: prevention of disease by personal and non-personal measures; care of patients who require investigation and treatment; and care of the sick who are not thought to need active intervention. Medical interest and resources are focused on the second area and, to a lesser extent, on personal prevention by immunization; the other responsibilities are relatively neglected.

The immediate determinant of the traditional range of interests is the patient's demand for acute care and the physician's wish to provide it. But the approach rests also on a conceptual model, on the belief that health depends primarily on intervention in disease processes.

This concept is not in accord with past experience. The improvement of health during the past three centuries was due essentially to provision of food, protection from hazards, and limitation of numbers.

Assessment of the determinants of human health (Chapter 7) suggests that the same influences are likely to be effective in future; but there is this difference, that in developed countries personal behaviour (in relation to diet, exercise, tobacco, alcohol, drugs, etc.) is now even more important than provision of food and control of hazards. According to this interpretation few diseases, except for an ill-defined group at the end of life, are determined irreversibly at fertilization; most congenital abnormalities are probably due to intra-uterine conditions operating during implantation and early embryonic development; and most other common diseases are due to post-natal influences. Prenatal determinants are likely to be difficult to identify and control; those which are post-natal vary widely, from some which are simple and tractable (as in the case of many infections) to others which are complex and difficult (for various reasons) to remove. Nevertheless it is on recognition of such influences that hopes for a solution of the problems of the common diseases, both physical and mental, largely rest.

Nothing in these conclusions suggests that the traditional lines of medical research are no longer needed. They have contributed greatly, by extending the scope and precision of hygienic measures, by immunization and therapy, and by providing an understanding of the body and its diseases on which the security of effective measures, originally largely intuitive, now substantially rests. However, there is need for a shift in the balance of effort, in recognition that improvement in health is likely to come in future, as in the past, from modification of the conditions which lead to disease, rather than from intervention in the mechanism of disease after it has occurred.

In health services the provision of acute care will continue to be predominant, needless to say, for it is a response to what the patient usually considers to be his most urgent need. But this service does not justify the place it has occupied until now in medical thought and practice. It is sometimes extremely effective; but often it is ineffective, or merely tides the patient over a short illness, leaving the underlying disease condition and prognosis essentially unchanged. The limitations of the traditional concept of the medical role would have been recognized much earlier, if health had not been transformed in the past three centuries by other influences.

What is needed is an adjustment in the balance of interest and resources between the three main areas of service referred to above. It is essential to give sufficient attention to the personal and non-personal influences which are the major determinants of health: to food and the environment, which will be mainly in the hands of specialists, and to personal behaviour, which should be the concern of every practising doctor. These interests should no longer be peripheral to the medical role, in the way that health education, nutrition, and environmental medicine have been peripheral hitherto. In the field of personal care, the making of a diagnosis and provision of acute care should be regarded as the beginning of a responsibility which will continue so long as the patient is unwell; and the arbitrary and largely artificial distinctions between different types of patients (acute, chronic, mental, subnormal, etc.) should end.

Index

Abdominal obstruction, 108
Abortion, 16, 22, 25, 43, 71, 73, 108–9, 167–8, 171, 192; spontaneous, 14, 24, 81
Abscess, 55
Accidents, 21, 169, 174, 183; death by, 83, 86, 181; treatment of, 108, 133, 175, 180, 187
Aetiology of disease, 12–14, 55, 117, 149; problems of interpretation, 19, 21, 25
Affluence, health and, viii, 11, 65, 81, 82, 83–7, 88–90, 120, 167, 168–71, 182, 183–4
Aged sick, the, 10, 137, 145, 154, 195; diseases of, 15–16, 25–44 passim, 89, see also 'Old age'
Agricultural life, 9, 71, 74–5, 80, 117, 161–2
Agricultural revolution, 6, 45, 63–5, 74, 75, 89, 117, 159, 182
Alcohol, consumption of, 67, 86, 126, 170, 180, 183
Amniocentesis, 181
Amyotrophic lateral sclerosis, xii
Anemia, 108
Anencephalus, 81
Anesthesia, 108
Antibiotics, 47, 50, 53, 54, 55, 77, 96–8, 105, 179, 185; misuse of, 187
Antitoxin, 47, 52, 77, 98–9, 102
Appendicitis, 37–8, 54, 77

Arthritis, 168, 173; osteo-, 113, 173
Asbestos, 170
Asthma, 42, 67
Atrial septal defect, 109
'Atrophy', 42, 66
Auto-immune diseases, 180; see also Eczema, Nephritis

BCG vaccination, 93–4, 106
Behaviour: modification of, 21, 69, 70, 72, 77–8, 79, 82, 87, 89–90, 118–19, 125–30, 144, 165, 169–71, 172, 173–4, 184; reproductive, 7, 9, 16, 43, 69, 70, 79, 87, 89, 160–1, 183–4; role of, viii, xv, 7–8, 9, 86, 89–90, 118–21, 125, 131, 144–6, 151, 172, 183, 197–8; science, technology and, 158, 160–1
Beaver, M.W., 58
Beri-beri, 62
Birthrates, see Fertility rates
Bovine infection, 53, 57
Breeding, selective, 6, 15, 165
Bronchitis, 24, 34–5, 41, 42, 50–1, 56, 96–8, 170
Burnet, Sir Macfarlane, 156–7, 179, 180–1

Cancer, 12, 39–40, 66, 85, 86–7, 88, 165–6, 171, 173; breast, 87, 129, 133, 139, 140, 174, 177, 183; cervical, 185; diagnosis of, 12, 124–5,

199

*Separate entry for individual diseases